P9-CTB-253

WITHDRAWN
No longer the property of the
Boston Public Library.
Sale of this material benefits the Library.

TICKED

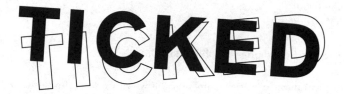

TICKED

A MEDICAL MIRACLE, A FRIENDSHIP,

AND THE WEIRD WORLD OF

TOURETTE SYNDROME

JAMES A. FUSSELL and JEFFREY P.MATOVIC

Foreword by JEFF FOXWORTHY

CHICAGO
REVIEW
PRESS

Copyright © 2013 by James A. Fussell and Jeffrey P. Matovic
Foreword copyright © 2013 by Jeff Foxworthy
All rights reserved
First edition
Published by Chicago Review Press, Incorporated
814 North Franklin Street
Chicago, Illinois 60610
ISBN 978-1-61374-380-5

Library of Congress Cataloging-in-Publication Data
Fussell, James A.
  Ticked : a medical miracle, a friendship, and the weird world of Tourette syndrome /
James A. Fussell with Jeffrey P. Matovic ; foreword by Jeff Foxworthy. — First edition.
    pages cm
  Summary: "An inspirational tale of personal struggle with and triumph over Tourette
syndrome, this is the story of Jeff Matovic and the radical treatment he sought to cure
himself. After suffering from Tourette's for years—with his tics and outbursts getting
progressively worse and with no results coming from drugs or physical or spiritual therapy—Jeff was able to convince his doctors and his insurance company to try a risky deep
brain stimulation treatment, a surgery that involves the implantation of a pacemaker for
the brain into his skull. Penned by a journalist who is also afflicted with Tourette's, this
is the incredible story of a friendship that blossomed under their common experiences
with this bizarre brain disorder. A complete discussion of the latest medical research of
and treatments for Tourette's, written in accessible and easy-to-understand terminology,
is also included"— Provided by publisher.
  ISBN 978-1-61374-380-5 (hardback)
  1. Matovic, Jeffrey P.—Health. 2. Fussell, James A.—Health. 3. Tourette syndrome—
Patients—United States—Biography. 4. Tic disorders—Patients—United States—Biography. I. Matovic, Jeffrey P. II. Title.

  RC375.F87 2013
  616.8'3—dc23

                              2012046321

Interior design: PerfecType, Nashville, TN

Printed in the United States of America
5 4 3 2 1

— For anyone who's ever had an impossible dream —

WE ARE PROFOUNDLY grateful and indebted to the late Dr. Robert Maciunas (1955–2011) for his incredible skill and intelligence, his enduring commitment and creativity, and his remarkable sensitivity and empathy. Consistently he went far beyond what was required of him, as a doctor and a man, to both save and change the lives of his patients. Personally and professionally, he was a shining example of hard work, stunning achievement, and all that is good in the world. Jeff and I hold him in the highest regard, and are honored and humbled to dedicate this book to his memory.

Contents

Foreword

Jeff Foxworthy

I KNOW WHAT it's like to walk into a room and have people stare at you—to see someone nudge and whisper something to the person next to them and then have the two turn and not-so-discreetly check you out. It's uncomfortable. I often have wished that I could just blend in. I imagine that must be a little of what it feels like to have Tourette Syndrome.

The difference is that I brought it on myself. And don't get me wrong; I love being a stand-up comedian. But comedians by nature are observers. We aren't very comfortable with being the observed. We want to get to know people's stories because within them are the common threads that tie us all together, and that is where the comedy lives.

I "met" Jim Fussell while doing a phone interview with the *Kansas City Star* newspaper to promote an upcoming live show I had in the area. It was the last interview in a string of five and was scheduled to last twenty minutes. Jim asked good questions, and I tried to provide entertaining, honest answers. We hit it off right from the get-go. As the interview progressed I starting asking him questions, looking for that common thread. It was then that he told me that he had Tourette Syndrome.

To be honest, I wasn't exactly sure what Tourette Syndrome was. I thought it was a disease that made you shout obscenities at random moments. In fact, I have a friend who talks in a very "colorful" language when he gets excited, and we have often jokingly accused him of having Tourette's. But as my grandmother used to say, "You are never too old to learn." So I asked Jim what Tourette's was—exactly? After all, we had been talking for a good half hour, and he had yet to shout a cuss word.

Jim explained that Tourette Syndrome was a misfiring of signals in the brain that caused a variety of afflictions or tics. Some people did indeed shout obscenities, while others might suddenly snap their head or flail an arm or leg. One lady had impulses to undress strangers. The comedian in me pondered that one for more than a moment. He told me that while there was no real cure, he had met a man who had symptoms so severe that he had risked his life to have a surgery that involved deep brain stimulation, and that his tics had disappeared. To be more accurate, they had been controlled.

This incredible man's name is Jeff Matovic. Jim found out about him after personally interviewing Oprah Winfrey. Jeff had appeared on an episode of *Oprah* and explained the horrors of this wicked disease and his life-changing surgery. Jim knew at that moment that he had to meet this miracle man.

And he did. And they talked. And Jim learned that when Jeff's tics were at their worst and his body ached so much that he wasn't sure if he would live through the hour, that the only way he could find relief was to listen to one of my comedy records.

"What? You've got to be kidding me!" I said. "And you and I are talking now?" This was starting to get weird. Our twenty-minute interview was now past the hour mark and I had no intention of hanging up the phone. I was fascinated.

"Jim," I said. "You have to tell this story." It was then that he mentioned that he had started writing a book about it, and asked if I would like to read an early draft. "Absolutely" I said, and a week later it arrived.

I read it in one sitting. It is a courageous piece of work. Jim has opened a door to a room that most people had no idea existed. He tells his story in conjunction with Jeff's story and he tells it with honesty. It is a story of frustration and hopefulness, a story of embarrassment and dignity, a story of great pain and of miraculous success. And within their story is the story of all of us—our desire not to be a freak or a weirdo, but to just be a man or a woman who is loved and accepted.

After reading the book I knew I had no choice but to call Jeff Matovic. When he answered the phone I said, "Jeff, this is Jeff Foxworthy" and there was a momentary silence. "Oh my gosh!" he said. "There were moments when you saved my life."

My eyes immediately welled up with tears. I was just trying to make people laugh. Saving someone's life had never factored into the equation. As we talked for a half hour I was overwhelmed with this man's faith, compassion, and goodness. After spending decades in pain and ridicule he had zero bitterness, only joy. His only desire was to encourage others.

When I hung up I thought about our conversation. I would never want the hand that either he or Jim had been dealt, but I hoped that if I had, I would handle it with half the grace and fortitude these two have shown. See, when you get to know the story of someone with Tourette Syndrome, you might stare at them when they walk into a room, but no longer out of morbid curiosity. It would be a stare of utter admiration.

This book is about more than one miracle man. It is about two of them, and then again it is about a million of them. It is about everyone with an affliction or deformity, everyone bald from the ravages of chemotherapy, everyone using a wheelchair or a walker. It is the story of each of us and of our quest for normalcy when in fact no one is normal. It is the story of our common humanity.

Thank you, Jim and Jeff, for your bravery in sharing your story with all of us. And may each of us leave this story with a new understanding and expanded compassion for others. You are heroes to all who know you.

God Bless.

Author's Note

Jim Fussell

IF I'VE LEARNED anything from being a newspaper reporter for nearly thirty years, it's this: our lives are jigsaw puzzles, and the pursuit of happiness nothing more than the search for their missing pieces.

This book is about just such a search. At its heart it's about how a thirty-year-old Cleveland man named Jeff Matovic tried to engineer his own recovery from one of the worst cases of Tourette Syndrome doctors had ever seen. For years his complex neurological tics worsened, leaving him suicidal. Desperate but determined, he latched onto one final chance—groundbreaking and experimental surgery that had never completely worked on someone with Tourette's.

For Jeff, finding a doctor courageous enough to attempt the operation meant a chance at a new life. For me—a person who has had Tourette's for nearly fifty years—finding Jeff meant finding a piece of my own puzzle that I was convinced didn't exist.

And that's really the point. This book is about more than just Jeff, or surgery, or Tourette Syndrome. It's about every person who's looking for a puzzle piece they've all but given up on finding. I am convinced there are pieces to fit all our puzzles; the trick is to never stop looking. That's as close as I can come to understanding the meaning of life. I truly believe we've all been put on this planet to work on our personal puzzles, and to help others work on theirs.

This story can help you with that. It is by turns impossible and inspiring. It will make you care and help you believe.

There's a reason why you picked up this book. Perhaps you needed to laugh, or cry. Maybe you needed a little emotional fuel to keep you going. Or maybe, like me, you just needed to realize that the pieces you seek to complete the puzzles in your life are possible to find.

Just remember, miracles *do happen*. And even when all seems lost, there is a reason to keep going.

It's called hope.

Author's Note

Jeff Matovic

> *"A moment's insight is sometimes worth a life's experience."*
>
> —Oliver Wendell Holmes

I'VE DISCOVERED SEVERAL intriguing facts in my life, some through self-exploration and others by sheer coincidence. Either way, they have been great teachers of life lessons.

- Celebrate life's' small victories.
- Fight for what you want and take it! Life will not always hand it to you.
- Create a visible blueprint to guide you to your goals.
- Maximize your potential.
- Embrace change.
- Don't limit yourself.
- The moment you think you can't go a step farther is often the exact moment when there is the biggest reward on the other side.
- Never allow someone else to define the parameters of your life.

But it wasn't until 2004 that I realized how much my relentless pursuits would pay off. And the truth of my effort rolled over me like a

steamroller as I lay awake on an operating table with a world-class neurosurgeon rooting around in my brain. I discovered that the impossible
was indeed possible after all, and ever since that day I've lived a life I
thought never existed—a normal one.

Whoever you are, you will find yourself in this book—and something for yourself in this book. This book is about the relentless pursuit
of what many of us cannot explain. Page by page, you'll find yourself
on a journey—a journey through the brightest of days and the darkest,
coldest nights. You'll find yourself searching for hope—and find that
there *is* hope—and wondering, laughing, and crying. And then you'll
find a young man giving life one more shot even though he had lost
belief in medicine, people, promises, treatments . . . and himself.

More than that, this book is about journeys, dreams, reality, confusion, love, and trying to find one's self and our fit in this world. Life
presents challenges every day. And sometimes we beg for nothing more
than a level playing field.

Whether you're an overstressed nine-to-five marketing manager; a
healthy, strong construction worker; or a parent who has had to hurdle
obstacles, make tough decisions, and seek an answer you just can't seem
to find, allow this book to inspire and bring a happy tear to your eye. It's
filled with the full spectrum of emotions.

It is my sincere hope that some of the things I've shared with you
will help guide you in your paths, travels, and adventures—wherever
they may take you.

1

Where's My Miracle?

*"Who then can so softly bind up the wound of another
as he who has felt the same wound himself?"*
—Thomas Jefferson

IN THE WINTER of 2004, in the features department of the *Kansas City Star*, I crawled under my messy, metal desk and began to sob. I didn't want to die. I just wasn't sure I had the strength to go on living. It was as if, when I wasn't looking, someone had reached into my chest and stolen all the hope out of my heart.

That's what Tourette Syndrome will do to you.

For forty years it had been a part of me, an evil puppet master forcing me to shake my head and twist my neck. And one dreary February morning, it simply overwhelmed me. The noises bouncing around the newsroom hit my head like a hammer. I wanted to disappear, to melt into the background. I slouched in my gray office chair and slowly began to sink. I had done this before. All the other times I caught myself and bolted upright. Not this time. I just ... kept ... going. Sliding off the front cushion of my chair, I plopped onto the coffee-stained carpet squares and pretended to look through some of my old stories that I kept on the floor in cardboard boxes. I liked the darkness and the snug feeling of protection. All of a sudden I was a child again, hiding in a fort, or under a blanket.

I was safe. But the feeling only lasted so long. In minutes the familiar urges to shake and move came back. I leaned over, resting my head against a stack of Sunday magazines, and closed my eyes until tears dripped from my short brown goatee. As a feature writer for nearly twenty years I couldn't count the number of times I had listened to other people pour out their problems—alcohol, drugs, depression, cancer, car accidents, financial ruin. The one constant was that everything always turned out for the best. There was a comfort to the form. The hurting person found a way to survive—even, in many cases, to prosper. I always felt good for them. I really did.

Except . . . where was *my* miracle?

One day I was just going to snap. And all it would take was three little words.

"How are you?" someone would ask at just the wrong time, and that would do it. I'd spin them around as they walked past.

"How am I?" I'd say, breathing a little too hard. "Not very good, thanks. I got two hours' sleep last night on top of one the night before. I feel like I'm carrying a three-hundred-pound man on my shoulders. My neck is on fire, and being stabbed by a thousand tiny ice picks. I'm so tired I can barely stand up, I can't remember my computer password, and I couldn't tell you what I wrote yesterday if you threatened to boil me in oil. My head is shaking, my neck is twisting, my stomach is tightening, and I worry that one of these mornings one of the monstrously hard head shakes I never let you see will finally jar something loose in my brain, and I'll pitch forward in my oatmeal and that'll be it for me. But thanks for asking. How are you?"

But then that would be wrong, wouldn't it?

Usually I just say I'm fine.

Back under my desk I shook my head so hard I banged my dollar-store reading glasses into the side of a metal drawer, mangling them into a shape that no longer fit my face. I took them off and tried to bend the flimsy metal frame back to something resembling straight.

A plastic lens fell out of the right side and wouldn't snap back in. *Whatever*, I thought. It was a perfect metaphor for my life. Bent up and broken, unable to be fixed. *That's* what more than forty years of Tourette Syndrome had done to me.

That also was the great irony of my life: the man who wrote about other people's happy endings who couldn't find one for himself.

Or could I?

As I sat hopeless and crying under my desk, there was something I didn't know. I didn't know that halfway across the country, at roughly the same time, a Cleveland neurosurgeon was pointing a spinning drill bit at a patient's head. I didn't know that he and another doctor had taken months to plot an elegant route through that patient's malfunctioning brain. And I certainly didn't know that patient was about to change my life in ways no one could have foreseen.

But he was.

And all I had to do was hang on long enough to find him.

2

Second Chance

"Courage is not the absence of fear, but rather the judgment that something else is more important than fear."

—Ambrose Redmoon

University Hospitals, Cleveland, Ohio. February 9, 2004, 9:30 AM.

The surgical-grade bone drill gave a throaty wail as its razor-sharp bit spun up to speed inches above Jeff Matovic's head. He knew its job; bore holes in his skull—two of them, nickel-sized, stopping just short of his brain.

Strapped to a padded operating table, head immobilized in a V-shaped titanium halo, the thirty-one-year-old closed his eyes and tried to breathe. He focused on the good things—his world-class doctors, the possibility of a new life, and the opportunity to advance research and make medical history. Sure, the operation had never worked on someone like him. But there was always a first time. Besides, he reminded himself, he'd asked for this. *Begged for it.*

No, risky, groundbreaking, quarter-million-dollar brain surgery wasn't something to dread. It was a second chance at life. And even if it didn't help him, he thought, maybe it would help someone else—later.

For three decades the six-foot-five Cleveland man struggled with a worsening case of the baffling movement disorder Tourette Syndrome. Sharp, repetitive, involuntary muscle spasms caused him to jerk like a mishandled marionette. There was no cure. No escape. Over thirty years, if he'd learned one thing about his condition it was this: severe Tourette's didn't kill you, it just made you *wish* you were dead.

He had tried prayer, pharmacies full of medications, even suicide. Now, staring into a bank of white-hot lights, he had one last hope.

Try for a miracle.

He dreamed of doing the little things other people took for granted—walking, talking, or holding blissfully still while doing *absolutely nothing*. He envisioned being well and getting the last laugh on every classless jackass who ever teased him, doubted him, or made his already hard life just a little harder.

At the same time he also remembered his maternal grandpa. He could still see the compassion in the old man's eyes when—unable to fight back an avalanche of tics—the tortured teen would begin to cry. His grandpa never told him to stop. Instead he'd remove his glasses and sob alongside the grandchild he so loved but couldn't fix.

"Jeff," he'd say, wiping his eyes. "I promise you they're going to find something someday."

Maybe, Jeff thought, *that someday is today.* But even he knew the odds were against him.

Years ago his mother had asked him a question: "What do you want out of your life?"

"Mom," he said. "I've had this so long that I really don't care that much about me anymore. I just want other people to be OK. I want kids like me to be able to go through grade school and not be made fun of. I want people to be able to walk through a mall or a street or a strip plaza and not have to worry about who's looking at them."

Weeks before surgery, he thought about that conversation as he wrote a letter to his doctors.

"Whatever happens in surgery," he told them, "whether I make it or not, I authorize you to audio tape, videotape, or use anything you can from this to help others."

In the waiting room his parents prayed their son would just make it through the operation alive.

Back on the operating table Jeff glanced to the side, past a blue surgical hood covering his head, to see a familiar face sporting gray hair, light green scrubs, and a gold chain. "How ya doing, doc?" he said, greeting his neurosurgeon.

"Doing fine," his surgeon said. "How are *you* doing?"

"I'm doing great," Jeff said, managing a smile. "Let's get this show under way."

Doctors had given him a local anesthetic and marked two spots, four inches apart, on his closely shaved head where the holes would be drilled (clearly). Unlike other surgeries, this one required him to be awake so he could give critical feedback to doctors as they implanted two electrodes deep in his brain.

The procedure was not new. It had helped patients with Parkinson's, dystonia, and essential tremor. But Tourette's was more complex, its vexing variety of symptoms nowhere near as well understood. The surgery was more than experimental. By all accounts, using a brain stimulator to try to interrupt the misfiring signals of Tourette Syndrome was a medical Hail Mary.

Maybe that's why no doctor had ever recommended it, or told him it had much of a chance to work. Worse, the operation wasn't even approved for Tourette's and carried risks of serious complications including stroke, paralysis, blindness—and death. The chance of death was small, less than 1 percent. But taken together, the risk of serious complications topped 20 percent.

Jeff didn't care. The way he saw it, he didn't have a choice. Enduring more in a day than many did in a lifetime, he'd lost interest in making it though one hellish day just to face another.

The drill wailed again.

Breathe, he told himself.

Louder now. It crept toward him.

This is what you wanted. This is your time.

He felt the bit tap against the top of his skull.

"Hold on with me, Jeff," his surgeon yelled over the racket. "You're going to feel a lot of pressure now."

As he saw little white bits of bone fly past his face, it felt like someone had dropped a house on his head. He closed his eyes as his body trembled, and he balled his hands into fists.

Hail Mary, full of grace.

3

Umm . . . Are You Taking My Clothes Off?

FOURTEEN YEARS BEFORE Tourette's drove me under my desk and caused Jeff to beg doctors to bore into his brain, I stood in the middle of a nine-floor atrium in McLean, Virginia, wondering if it was illegal to be naked in the lobby of a Hilton hotel.

I know. What does one have to do with the others?

Everything.

In many ways this is where my part of the story starts. My wife, Susan, and I attended the 1990 National Conference of the Tourette Syndrome Association as delegates from Kansas City. This is where I first *really* learned about Tourette's—and myself. More important, it is a key link in the chain of events that got me my job in the features department of the *Kansas City Star*, which led me to a face-to-face meeting with Oprah Winfrey, which led me to Jeff and the improbable miracles that helped change my life.

And it all started with a slender brunette in a little black dress.

"I'm Jennifer," she said, kissing me softly on my cheek. "And I have to do this."

Working quickly she unbuttoned my shirt to my navel, then pressed her cold hand flat against my warm chest.

A lot goes through your mind when a beautiful stranger suddenly starts unbuttoning your shirt. On the one hand, it was sexy as hell. On the other, it was sad. Her hands said one thing; her eyes quite another.

I smiled nervously and looked around for my wife.

"This is embarrassing," Jennifer said, yanking my shirttail out of my trousers as if trying to start a pull-cord lawn mower. "But you've got to understand. It's just what I do."

You . . . molest people? I thought.

"I can't help it," she said in a small voice. "I just can't help it."

I knew that. None of the people I met that day could help it. Tourette's is like a tornado that rages through your body. It leaves behind a debris field of unwanted movements and bizarre behaviors. They crop up in the most amazing ways; in tics and twitches, outbursts and compulsions, and—in the most extreme form—in Jeff Matovic's unendurable spasms.

The conference offered information, education, and support. But now, it seemed, I was the entertainment. A group of onlookers who knew Jennifer liked to unbutton things was now deriving great pleasure from seeing her unbutton me. I didn't know what to do. I didn't know what to say. I didn't even shake. I just froze like a semi-naked statue. As I stood there Jennifer moved to my left and applied breathy butterfly kisses to my check and neck. As I grew progressively unclothed, more people began to stare. I knew I had to stop her, but it was getting hard to think. I held up my right index finger as I searched for a word, but all that came out was "Uhhh."

Jennifer was in her early twenties and quite attractive. I was in my early thirties and quite married. I scanned the crowd, looking for a strawberry blonde head of hair—always the easiest way to spot my wife.

Oh God, I thought. *What's Susie going to think of* this?

Then I remembered. It was almost ten, and she had gone back up to the room to rest.

So far I had met a handful of people with varying types and severities of Tourette's. One of my favorites was Bob, a young man with wire-rimmed glasses and curly black hair who looked like he'd swallowed a Michelin truck tire. Every few seconds Bob would fling his right arm out and flick his wrist as if shooting an imaginary foul shot. Recently diagnosed with Tourette's, he had driven ten-straight hours to get to the conference.

That night we traded stories until after midnight in the hotel bar. We'd talk, then Bob would pause to take a shot.

It was nice. I even took a couple of shots myself.

Bob didn't mind.

The people in the bar—and I include myself in this—reminded me a bit of the famous cantina scene in the original *Star Wars*. It was there, at the spaceport of Mos Eisley, that moviegoers first learned of the odd and startling collection of characters that lived in that galaxy. It was the same feeling for me as I learned about the equally odd and startling collection of characters who struggled with Tourette Syndrome.

In one corner, a dark-haired man wearing a Yankees cap sat at a table and slapped himself repeatedly in the face. After every slap he'd readjust his cap, which he'd knocked cockeyed on his head. Then he'd say "I dare you to do that again!"

Vibrating like an unbalanced washer, he'd grimace and stare straight ahead as if fighting off his inner demons before exploding with another slap to his face. When a friend joined him at the table, the man reached out, as if in desperation, to grasp his hand. He held on tightly with his slapping hand and didn't let go. After that, the slapping stopped.

In another corner, a woman with long curly hair the color of strained peaches seemed oddly fascinated by the game Duck, Duck, Goose. She shook and twitched like I did, only worse. When her head snapped, her shoulder-length hair flew as if she were in a wind tunnel. Then she'd go into her rap.

"Duck, duck, *GOOOOOOOOOOOOOOO—SE*," she'd say, yelling the goose part as loudly as she could. As she did she turned her gaze to the ceiling like a wolf howling at a full moon.

Then there were the people who swore. You heard it intermittently throughout the hotel, usually forced out as if the words were breaking out of some sort of linguistic prison. *Fuck* and *fucker* were the most common, although *cocksucker* wasn't far behind. Sometimes people would shout the words repeatedly, almost musically, as they bobbed their head. Some got pretty good at it, and I came to respect their sense of timing and rhythm. Other times the profanities came unbidden in the middle of an otherwise normal conversation, such as the one I had with a nattily dressed man with a Middle Eastern accent.

"Hi, how are you?" he said, catching my eye at a reception in the lobby.

"Fine, thanks," I responded. "You?"

"Good. Can't complain."

"I'm Jim," I said, extending my hand. "I'm from Kansas City."

"I'm John, and I'm from—YOU FUCKING COCKSUCKER!—Chicago."

I think that's why I stuck close to Bob. I was still new to this more intense form of Tourette's. And after being undressed, cursed at, and watching people hit themselves in the face, a man who shot free throws seemed a little more my speed.

When I had to go, Bob thanked me for the conversation.

"You don't know how it is to have felt so weird all these years, like you're the only one who does these strange things," he said.

I wrenched my neck hard to the right and blinked my eyes.

"Then again," he said, "I guess you do."

— —

WITH NO MORE buttons to undo, Jennifer's long index finger traced a playful line down my right cheek, then dropped straight to my belt buckle. At one point her hand came dangerously close to heading straight down Broadway.

"*Hell-o,*" I said, jumping back as if someone had dropped a firecracker at my feet. "You *are* a friendly one, aren't you?"

I wanted to be sensitive. But then Jennifer began pawing at the zipper of my pants. I politely guided her hand away and excused myself.

"It was very nice meeting you, but I . . . think I better find my wife."

You learn a lot going to a Tourette Syndrome conference. The first thing I learned is you have to be ready for anything.

"*Aaaauuuughhhhhhhh!*"

I flinched as a terrifying scream echoed through the room over my right shoulder. Had someone been stabbed? Seen a dead body? I turned toward the sound in time to see a middle-aged man with tufts of graying hair around his temples just finishing his yell. I didn't get his name, but I'll never forget the sound. It came out of nowhere every few minutes as he talked, a bloodcurdling blast that seemed to come from the depths of his tortured soul. An articulate and well-informed speaker, he seemed particularly interested in history and foreign policy. When his symptom came he simply excused himself by holding his right index finger in the air in front of his mouth as if to say "one second."

Then he turned his head and screamed as if Hannibal Lecter had jumped from behind a pillar with some fava beans and a nice Chianti. Seconds later he resumed his talk, without explanation, exactly where he had left off.

Even though I had been diagnosed in 1984, it was here at the conference that I first saw proof that there were others like me in the world—otherwise normal people whose bodies did things beyond their control. And it was on that night that I realized that Tourette Syndrome was one of the most fascinating conditions I had ever seen. Sure, other conditions were more serious. Some of them were killers. But when it came to personality, they were pretty much one-trick ponies. Diabetes? MS? Cancer? Compared to them Tourette's was the funhouse mirror of maladies. The same disease that made me shake my head and blink my eyes made Jennifer unbutton shirts and a middle-aged man scream like Janet Leigh in the shower.

The word *odd* hardly did it justice.

Tourette's is thought to be caused by a chemical imbalance in the brain. Or, in some cases, researchers think, it might be due to an abnormality in a certain chromosome that broke off and reattached itself backward. Estimates of how many suffer from the syndrome vary widely. Some experts claim that about one hundred thousand people in this country have full-blown cases. Others, counting mild cases that likely go unreported, say the number could be in the millions. But the numbers are nowhere near as dramatic as the variety of physical and vocal tics, odd behaviors, thoughts, and compulsions the disorder spawns. It may cause you to blink your eyes, blurt out swear words, howl like a banshee, hop like a bunny rabbit, have racing thoughts, unbutton people's shirts, or repeat the last word of a sentence endlessly— endlessly, endlessly.

Or it may cause you to shake your head as I do.

There is no cure for Tourette Syndrome, but some drugs can lessen the severity of its symptoms. Researchers believe that in some cases Tourette Syndrome is genetic, and there is evidence that it runs in families, although not in mine.

My Tourette's was mild in comparison to others' at the conference. But it was bad enough. Since it wasn't always obvious, some other delegates asked me about my symptoms.

So I told them.

Ever since I was young, I said, I've felt an impossible-to-describe tension in my body. It's a constant, anxious uneasiness. But even that's not a good description. There just aren't any words that do it justice. Whatever it is, it's always building, worsening. The tide is coming in. Sometimes it comes in gentle ripples, other times in larger waves. And sometimes it's a tsunami. Whether it takes two seconds or two hours, eventually the urges becomes so strong that it's impossible to focus on anything else. At such a time the only three things I care about are getting rid of the feeling, getting rid of the feeling, and getting rid of the feeling. And the only way to do that is by ticking, which in my case means wrenching my neck or shaking my head in a certain way until it feels right. Even if the relief only lasts a few seconds, it's worth it.

I told them about the time former singer and orange juice spokeswoman Anita Bryant said she could cure me in her hotel room. I told them about the time I ran in circles in a parking lot at midnight in snow up to my calves after a bad reaction to a medicine. I told them about the time I shrieked in the streets like a banshee, the time I had to stay home from school for two months during second grade, and the time my own father told me to stop it because I was shaking like a chicken with its head cut off.

But more on that later.

The point is, when I told the stories to stranger after stranger they nodded their heads. They knew all too well what I was talking about.

Back home, almost nobody knew.

Trying to tell someone who doesn't have Tourette's about it is like trying to teach trigonometry to a ten-year-old. You can do it, but only to a point. One of my neighbors even said "You're making that up" before realizing I was serious.

A lot of people are fooled by Tourette's. Just ask all the doctors in Pennsylvania or Nebraska who failed to diagnose me with a single medical problem. Or my father, who was a PhD and a voracious reader. Or my mother, who had a master's degree and worked as a newspaper reporter. Or my uncle Dick, a psychiatrist who first suggested I go talk to somebody. Or any of my neighbors or teachers or counselors or ministers or friends. Nobody knew why I shook and twitched—least of all me.

When I was a boy there were very few sources of information about people with Tourette's. There was no Internet, no support groups, no HBO specials, no books, associations, nor national conferences. But it could have been worse. I could have lived in the Middle Ages, where I can only imagine people with Tourette's were thought to be possessed by the devil. When not being flogged or burned as witches, they were likely confined to asylums. Such draconian treatments eventually disappeared.

Unfortunately they were replaced by ignorance of a different stripe. Well into the twentieth century the public and medical community thought children with tics were likely the result of abuse or bad parenting. Even in 1990 some doctors still misdiagnosed people with Tourette's as having psychological issues, epilepsy, or schizophrenia. More than one hundred years after the first case of Tourette Syndrome was described in 1885 by French neurologist Georges Gilles de la Tourette, you'd think all doctors would be familiar with Tourette's.

You'd be wrong. While my neurologist was a good source of information, several general practitioners I went to in the 1990s still knew nothing about it.

It's no wonder. Only eighteen years earlier, in 1972, the National Institutes of Health turned down a grant proposal by the newly formed Tourette Syndrome Association because the reviewers believed "there were probably no more than one hundred cases of Tourette's in the entire nation." Today, a website sponsored by the same National Institutes of Health and the US Library of Medicine, the largest medical library in the world, put the prevalence of all forms of Tourette's at roughly 1 percent of the population. That's three million people in the United States alone. And even that's a conservative estimate, since many people with mild tics usually don't seek medical attention.

Is there still misinformation about Tourette Syndrome today? You be the judge. On the forum page of something called Godlike Productions (www.godlike productions.com/forum1/message551803/pg1) the following question was up for discussion: "Is Tourettes [*sic*] syndrome demon posession [*sic*]?"

"Yes," wrote an anonymous poster from the United Kingdom. "In my humble opinion it is demon possession, and can be cured by an adept spiritual healer."

Then there was this response from Observer from Australia.

"Yes!! Tourette's is part possession. As some have stated it is the responsibility of the semi-possessed to learn to overcome. It is also in BLACK AND WHITE for the stupid to see!"

And, finally, there was this post by Grower from the United States.

"M I a bad person for laughing uncontrollably at people with this disease?"

No, Grower. Just an ignorant one. And you'd better hope with all your heart that comedian Ron White is wrong when he says "You can't fix stupid."

But I pray every day that they *can* fix people like me. They *are* working on it. Some researchers believe Tourette's may be a small key that unlocks a bigger door. An article in *Harvard Men's Health Watch* magazine put it this way:

> Tourette's is especially interesting to . . . scientists because its symptoms lie on the border between the voluntary and the involuntary, the physical and the mental, the normal and the pathological. A better understanding of these symptoms could lead to a better understanding of many other neurological and behavior disorders.

Honestly? At the time of the convention I didn't care about other people's neurological disorders. I just wanted to believe that I had a chance to get rid of mine. But more than that, I wanted to believe I was worth something, that I had a future, that my life could be more than just surviving. I was looking for some hope and some humanity in a disorder I could neither change nor understand. And despite being undressed, screamed at, and cursed out a thousand miles from home, I had found it.

In at least some way, every person I met at that hotel helped change my life for the better. But the person with Tourette's who would have the greatest impact on my life wasn't at that conference. He was still a junior in high school. But by that time he had already handled more serious problems than most people face in a lifetime.

One of his scariest challenges came in the fourth grade.

4

The Hand of Satan

"HOLY SHIT!"

Jeff mouthed the words under his breath as thunder rumbled outside his fourth-grade social studies classroom at St. Bonaventure Parish School in Glenshaw, Pennsylvania. With his hands folded in front of him he *tried* to pay attention to the no-nonsense nun saying something about the War of 1812. But all he could think about were the fingers of his right hand, which slowly had begun to tighten around the fingers of his left.

At first the prolonged squeezing was harmless as a handshake.

Then it started to hurt.

What was going on? Why was his hand squeezing like that?

He pulled, trying to free his left hand from the firm grip of his right—but couldn't.

And then it got worse. The powerful muscles in his right forearm, bicep, and shoulder doubled the strength of their flex, causing the fingers of his right hand to clench rigidly, as if in the throes of rigor mortis. This was not a hand anymore. It was a *weapon*!

"Ow!" he gasped, as his eyes darted around the room and out to the hallway to see if anyone had noticed.

He had done strange things before—blinked his eyes, hissed like a snake, and repeatedly cleared his throat. Habits he would outgrow, his mother assured him.

This was different.

For the first time his body not only rejected his will, but caused him physical pain. For the first time he felt like he wasn't in control. For the first time he started to think something was *seriously* wrong with him.

He moved his hands to his lap and jiggled them like a key in a lock. No change.

As lightning lit up the dreary sky the nine-year-old looked at his hands as if he'd never seen them before. His right hand was now squeezing so hard it had turned his badly swollen left hand a sickly white after pushing all the blood to the ends of his dark red fingertips. His heart beat faster and his breaths became labored as he thrashed in his seat.

Two minutes now. He had to do something—*fast*!

What if his right hand never let go? Would he crack his own bones? Would a doctor have to operate? He put both hands between his thighs and drew in his knees. He didn't know what to do. One thing he *did* know was that he couldn't stay there. He stood up suddenly and bolted out the door to the boys' restroom. His thoughts went quickly to Sister Joanne, the thin, black-haired, middle-aged teacher known as the strictest nun in school. You *did not* leave Sister Joanne's class without permission. Not unless you wanted to get sent to Father Ed.

He didn't have a choice.

In the bathroom he looked at his swollen left hand and felt sick. Three minutes. He could no longer feel his left hand, and part of his left forearm had gone numb as well. He struggled with the faucet but finally managed to turn on the cold water full blast. Desperate, he shoved his hands under the forceful stream, removing them only briefly to splash water awkwardly on his flushed face. The icy water splashed wildly—out of the sink, onto his pants, and all over the floor—but it did its job. The cold helped reduce the swelling enough to allow him to pull his hands apart.

Bruised and sore, his crumpled left hand had five blood red indentations where the fingernails of his right hand had dug far into his flesh. As the blood began to return, his hand started to throb and tingle. The pain was like nothing he had felt before. It was as if he had just removed his hand from his father's workshop vise.

With the water finally turned off, he looked at himself in the mirror. *What is wrong with you?* he thought.

Sister Joanne had sent one of Jeff's closest friends, Dan Kenaan, into the restroom to retrieve him. Dan, a slender, brown-haired boy about a half-foot shorter than Jeff, found his friend sitting in one of the toilet stalls with the door open, cradling his left hand like a wounded animal. By this time his right arm had grown so fatigued the contractions had stopped. For a moment the two boys stared at each other, saying nothing. Jeff looked down at his wet, red, and dripping hand, then extended it gently, as if to say "See?"

"I'll tell Sister Joanne you need to go to the nurse right away," Dan said.

Dan's instructions were to return immediately to class with Jeff. Instead he walked beside his friend, slowly across the length of the building, to the clinic.

When they got there Dan looked at Jeff.

"You OK?" he said.

"I'll be all right," Jeff said. "And you can tell Kevin I'm OK, too."

Dan nodded and walked back to class. After telling the nurse he had an upset stomach, Jeff called his mother and went home. He never told anyone what really happened.

JEFFREY PAUL MATOVIC was born on January 23, 1973, in Canton, Ohio. He was such a happy boy his mother called him her "Sunshine Baby." But it didn't take long for that sun to go under a cloud. By the time he was a toddler, doctors became concerned about how his legs were growing. The bones from his hips to his knees curved. Doctors fitted him with heavy steel braces that he wore twenty-three hours a day. Twenty buckles that were progressively tightened forced his bones to straighten, while an elastic strap running from one brace to the other forced his hip joints to open.

His father affectionately called his youngest "Buckle Boy."

The first day Jeff got his braces his mother carried him into the living room and deposited him on the floor next to his older brother. A short time later, Steve was impressed enough to call something to his parents' attention.

"Well, look at this big boy!" he said.

Jeff had flopped his left leg over his right, forcing him to roll onto his belly. Then he pushed on the floor with his hands and—for the first time with his new braces on—stood up by himself.

Although he hated them, Jeff wore the buckles faithfully. The one hour he didn't wear them came after his afternoon nap, when his mother let him run and play. When it was time to put them back on, he never ran from his mother.

But he always cried.

He had just learned to climb stairs and ride a tricycle. It broke his mother's heart. She just prayed it would do him some good.

His parents took Jeff to mass each week in a little red wheelchair to receive blessings from a priest. Six months later his doctor removed the braces, and Jeff's legs grew long and strong. He spent summer days racing with his friends through the streets of his suburban Pittsburgh neighborhood.

The sunshine was back!

At least for a while. Soon his parents began to notice odd sounds and behaviors. Their youngest would obsessively smell things, and hiss like a snake. Jeff knew something was wrong with him years before his diagnosis. Tears rolled down his cheeks nearly every morning while walking to first grade.

He still remembers his first tic. It was 1977 and he was a kindergartener in the Houston suburb of Spring, Texas, where his family had recently moved, following his father's work for the steel industry. He had just gotten out of the bath and was getting ready to pull on his Dallas Cowboys pajamas on a warm and humid night.

"Make sure you dry off completely, honey," his mother, Patty Matovic, called. "You don't want to stick to your PJs."

After brushing his teeth and combing his short black hair he looked in the mirror expecting to see himself staring back. Instead he saw a stranger making a series of odd facial grimaces. He watched in fascination and concern as his jaw involuntarily moved to the right, and then back to the left so hard it caused his eye to close. Over and over his lips puckered into a fish kiss as if he were a smallmouth bass. Then, just like that, it stopped.

"That was weird," he said with a shrug. "I guess today is just one of those funny days."

He had no idea what was to come.

Before long he was forcefully spreading the fingers of his hand apart as hard as he could.

"Relax," his father would say. "You're so fidgety."

Worried he would hurt himself, his mother gave him a large, rectangular wooden block to hold in an effort to keep his fingers occupied.

It didn't work.

That wasn't the only thing he did with his fingers. As a small boy he smelled them. Not like a normal child would smell something, but by jamming them—all of them—under his nose at the same time. He'd press them tightly against the opening of his nostrils, as if compelled by some unseen force. Then he'd take a sniff—a deep, long, lusty sniff that made a sound that could be heard halfway across his family's ranch house.

He'd smell other things, too—a dirty sock, a pencil, a fork, a piece of paper. As with his other habits, his pediatrician said he would outgrow it.

Jeff hated having to smell things. When he would smell his scissors at school his teacher would say, "Put those scissors on the desk! You're going to put your eye out!"

He put the scissors down, then sat on his hands to keep the confusing compulsion from making him smell them again. That was hardly any better. Soon after, his teacher would yell at him for not doing his work.

In another class a teacher would ask him, "Why are you blinking your eyes so much?

Jeff didn't just blink. He burst his eyelids as wide open as they would go, and thrust his eyeballs forward forcefully toward the ceiling as if trying to make them pop from his head. At the same time his head jerked back. Then he would slam his eyelids closed and his head would nod forward.

By fifth grade Jeff was taller than many of his teachers. Fast, strong, and coordinated, he could throw or kick a ball farther than anyone in school. But combined with his tics, his athleticism was too often explosive and off-putting. One time, while playing four square, he felt a sudden arm tic. Embarrassed, he threw the ball to make the tic look natural.

Afterward a girl told him he couldn't play anymore because they were afraid he'd throw the ball into the street.

He didn't know what to do. Often he would pretend to be sick and ask to go to the clinic. He would lie on a small bed as the nurse called his mother.

"What's wrong, sweetie?" his mother said in a soothing voice.

Tears rolled down his face. "I miss you and Dad," he said. "And I just want to come home."

The nurse would put a thermometer in his mouth. Sometimes he would cup his hands to his mouth and blow warm air to try to make the thermometer heat up.

It didn't work.

His mother consoled him.

"Jeffrey Paul, calm down," she'd say. "Take a cool cloth and wipe your face and just listen. Now that you've calmed down, I want you to stay at school. The school day will be over in a couple hours."

He *hated* that line. A couple hours? Was she crazy?

"Sometimes your dad doesn't feel like going to work. But sometimes you just need to hang in there." She had no idea how much he did—every day.

Home was better. But there were problems there too. Many mornings his father, Jim, heard the loud sniffing sound from the kitchen. The distracting sound made it hard to concentrate on the morning news coming from the radio that sat on the kitchen counter. "Why does he do that, Patty?"

Slender and athletic, Jim Matovic wore white shirts and dark pants to work at a company called Jones & Laughlin, where he worked with computers in the steel industry. He spent his day with facts and numbers, debugging codes and solving problems. He didn't like it all that much. But at least a string of computer code never sniffed so loudly it caused him to miss Paul Harvey.

"Well?" Jim Matovic said, taking a sip of his coffee.

Patty Matovic didn't know why her youngest son sniffed so violently, or why he sometimes hissed like a snake—or cleared his throat, blinked his eyes, kicked his leg, punched at nothing, or forcefully spread the fingers of his hand. He wouldn't talk about it. He made excuses, or changed the subject, or left the room.

So she just said what she always said, hoping it was true. "It's just a phase, honey," she'd say. "A habit. He'll grow out of it."

That was fine when Jeff was three. But now he was ten.

"LET'S GO! WHO'S got the ball?"

It took more than a week for Jeff's left hand to heal fully from the squeezing attack. As soon as it did he knew exactly what he wanted to do—play baseball with friends. In spring he played every day after school and on the weekends. And in summer he played almost every night.

Before the games his mother would mix up lime-green Kool-Aid—enough for the entire neighborhood—and boys on bikes would fill their school Thermoses with the jade-colored liquid. Then they'd grab their gloves and take the short ride up the hill to St. Bonnie's and play on the school's large faculty parking lot.

For Jeff, staying active helped stem the tide of the mysterious movements and obsessive compulsions gradually taking over inside his body. There was nothing like running, throwing, catching, hitting, and fielding to help take his mind off it for a couple of hours.

As summer flew by the strange urges only grew stronger. Until then he had hidden his movements, explained them away, changed the subject, or simply refused to talk about them. But as they started to combine and increase, he could avoid them no longer. One night, after a two-hour baseball game in late August, he asked Dan Kenaan and Kevin Keenan to stick around.

"You guys are my best friends in the whole world," he said, looking down. "So . . . I'm going to tell you something that nobody knows—*and don't tell anybody else, OK?*"

They nodded.

Jeff took a breath and blew it out. "You've seen how sometimes I, you know, move weird and stuff?"

He picked blades of grass and flicked pieces of gravel with his index finger as if kicking the extra point in a game of paper football. As he reclined in the grass his leg began to kick and twitch, causing his thigh muscles to convulse under his shorts, as if to music.

Not now! he thought. His heart sank. What would they say about this?

He knew what they'd say: "You know what, dude? You're a freak! Don't ask us to come back and play with you anymore!"

His eyes began to blink rapidly. He looked off to the left and expelled air rapidly from his lungs with a sharp *Huh! Huh!* sound.

"You OK, man?" Kevin said.

"Yeah . . . uh, yeah," Jeff said unconvincingly.

"Dude, it's cool," Kevin said. "Whatever it is, just tell us."

Jeff's tics were alive, with their own personality. As soon as they knew someone felt comfortable around them, they came out even stronger. And this was a green light to let 'er rip. Jeff's right arm began to punch, then his left. His eyes blinked and bulged out of their sockets, and his neck began to roll.

He steadied himself, then swallowed hard. "Those—*huh!* Those things I do in class when my arm and my neck move and you see me blink and stuff," he said. "I can't help that. And I don't want it to happen, 'cause it *hurts*."

"Dude, do your parents know about this?" said Kevin. "Your parents are awesome! They might even know what it is or help you."

"It ain't that easy," Jeff said. "I wanna be like everybody else. I don't want to be weird. I don't want to stand out anymore than I already do."

"What are you talkin' about?" said Dan.

"People—*Huh! Huh!*—people point and laugh."

"I'll beat 'em down!" said Kevin.

"Thanks, guys," Jeff said, almost out of breath. "Just don't tell anyone, OK? 'Cause I'm still trying to figure this out."

"No problem, man," Dan said.

When they got up off the grass, it was nearly 9:00 PM and growing dark. Kevin and Dan slung their bags of gear around their shoulders to head home.

Before getting on his bike, Kevin looked back at Jeff. "Dude, it's all right," he said. "We'll get through this."

"Yeah, whatever, man," Dan said. "Whatever you do it's not like we're not going to like you anymore."

Overcome with relief, Jeff grabbed Dan and lifted him high in the air, causing the balls and bats to tumble out of his bag. Then, using all the power in his nearly six-foot frame, he lifted Kevin and gave him a high five. "Thanks, guys," he said.

"All right, all right," said Dan, putting an end to the touchy-feely stuff. "Let's make a bet. See that sign?"

He pointed to a stop sign about thirty feet away.

"Yeah," Jeff said.

"Let's have some target practice."

Jeff looked at the sign in the distance and smiled. He nodded as
Dan flipped him an old scuffed baseball.

"Watch this," he said. He stared down the sign, then went into a
pitcher's windup. Then he fired the ball as hard as he could with a grunt.

"I just wish things would *stop!*" he said, emphasizing the last word
just as the ball clanged hard off the metal sign, leaving a baseball-sized
dent between the *T* and the *O.*

Then Dan threw.

"It's *gonna* stop!" he yelled, leaving another dent.

Then Kevin.

"It's *gotta* stop!"

Fifteen minutes later the sign was nearly facing the opposite
direction.

It was past nine, and past their curfew.

By this time, Jeff was nearly out of breath from the exertion he put
into his throws. "I think we got it, dude," Kevin said, heading for his
bike. "We better go."

"Wait," Jeff said. He ran to the pockmarked sign and turned it back
the right way.

"Cool?" he said, smiling and raising his open hand.

"Cool man," Kevin said, completing the high five.

5

The Tic Explosion

JEFF DIDN'T KNOW what was wrong with him until 1983.

He was ten years old.

The weekend that changed his life started innocently enough as he walked home from fifth grade with his older brother.

"Man, you got it comin' to you when we get home and play pool," said Jeff, who resembled a nearly six-foot-tall Beaver Cleaver. "You're *goin' down*!"

"Bring it on, little man," said Steve, who—at two years older—was a few inches taller.

"Whatever, Holmes."

When they reached their front yard they removed their backpacks and Jeff held the front door for his brother.

"Ladies and losers first," he said.

"Ahhh, shaddup," said Steve.

As they did most days after school, they headed to the ranch house's finished basement—the War Room, as they called it.

"Rack 'em, lady," Jeff said in advance of a game of Eight Ball.

"I might as well, 'cause I'll be breakin' once I win," said Steve.

Jeff and Steve were accomplished at pool, having played since they were tall enough to see over the side rail. Their father, who had played day and night while stationed at an air force base in Okinawa, taught them both pool and Ping-Pong.

Jeff drew back his stick and sent the cue ball rocketing forward in a white blur. The crack of the break echoed through the basement as he sent the blue ten ball rolling into a corner pocket.

"Stripes," he called.

The brothers traded shots and good-natured jabs until Jeff had only two balls left. He chalked his cue as the room grew quiet. Before he could shoot, his right arm flew from his side in an involuntary tic. He yawned and played it off as a stretch, then went back to his shot.

Although Jeff had ticked in front of his family before, he never talked about it. It was too embarrassing, too humiliating. He sooner would have lit himself on fire.

He sniffed and blinked, then pretended to blow his nose, covering his face with a handkerchief. Glancing at Steve out of the corner of his eye, he wondered how much he had seen, how much he knew. He bent over the shot again, half studying the angles and half wishing he could talk to his brother about the strange urges and compulsions threatening to tear him apart.

Jeff chalked his stick again as he stared straight ahead.

"*Today* would be nice," Steve said.

Jeff took a deep breath and blew it out. "Life's just not fair sometimes, is it?" he said.

Steve furrowed his brow. "It can be pretty brutal," he said. "Why do you bring that up?"

"Just lately a lot of stuff's been getting in my way, and it's a lot of stuff I can't control," Jeff said.

He shot, and missed.

"What are you getting at?" Steve asked as he walked around the table for his shot. "Is it girls? Is anyone treating you bad or messin' with ya?"

"No. Nothing like that. It's just a . . ."

"A what?" Steve shot and missed.

"It's just a shitty time for me right now," Jeff said. He looked away. "But let's just get on with the game."

In one way Jeff never wanted to have to talk about the strange things his body was doing. In another he almost wished Steve would ask him about them. He almost did months ago when they were walking home from school.

"School's goin' pretty good, huh?" Jeff said.

"Classes are pretty good, recess is awesome, lunch is average at best."

"For me things are going . . . fine," Jeff said, looking at the ground. "I guess." He kicked at stones and sticks on the pavement as he walked.

Steve stopped Jeff and grabbed him by the arm.

"Are things really OK, or are you just saying that?" he said.

Jeff couldn't look at his brother. He stared into the sky instead.

"You know," Steve said, "if you ever just need to tell me something, no matter what it is, you know that's cool with me."

"Yeah, I know," Jeff said, blinking back tears. He fidgeted with his shirt and adjusted his belt. The lump in his throat felt like a beach ball. "Things are . . . things are not as good as I'd want them to be."

— ⸰ —

THAT SUNDAY, IN the living room, Jeff and Steve watched the Miami Dolphins play the New England Patriots. "The Killer Bs are gonna sting these dudes!" Jeff said, using the popular nickname for the Dolphin defense, which had six starters with last names that started with *B*.

Steve got up from his recliner and left. Moments later he returned with a dead bee in his hand that he had been saving for a week.

"Here's your Killer B, numbskull!" he said, pushing the dead insect close to Jeff's face.

Jeff jumped off the couch as if Steve had poured hot coffee in his lap.

"You're sick!" he said, slapping Steve's hand. "Get that thing outta here!"

The bee fell onto the carpet by the coffee table.

"You better pick that up. Mom just vacuumed," Jeff said. He imitated his mother's stern voice. "*You better get that straight, Steven James*!"

"Yeah, yeah. Shut up."

Steve threw away the bee in the kitchen. When he returned he turned off the TV.

Jeff threw up his hands. "What'd you do that for?"

Steve held out a bright pink rubber football they called the Pinkie.

"Get your butt of that couch," Steve said. "We're gonna throw the ball."

In their large backyard Steve grabbed the Pinkie and lined up like a quarterback under center. Jeff lined up wide to his left like a receiver and waited for Steve to call the play. Jeff ran about a half dozen pass patterns before Steve called a play that called for Jeff to go deep.

Steve put a serious look on his face. He looked left and right as he placed his hands under an imaginary center and pretended to survey the defense.

"Forty-four, L, F, three-thirty-three, on two. Set. Hut *hut!*"

Jeff sprinted fifteen steps and cut hard left to fake an out route. After Steve pump faked, Jeff pivoted and exploded upfield.

This was Jeff's favorite play. The most exciting play. *The long bomb!*

"Elway back to pass," Steve called as Jeff sprinted across the emerald grass as fast as he could go. "Sees his man . . ."

Steve let the Pinkie fly in a high arcing spiral that seemed to hang in the sky forever.

Jeff looked into the high blue sky, his excitement building as he looked up and found the spinning ball. It was a perfect pass, and he was going to catch it. Then Steve was going to raise his arms and yell "Touchdown!"

And then it happened. Something weird. Something he didn't understand. Something he had never felt before. Suddenly, Jeff broke off his route and shook from head to heel. The ball sailed far over his head as he came to a standstill and kept shaking—hard arm and leg jerks accompanied by a series of deep knee bends and the rapid exhalation of air.

"*Huh! Huh!*" he grunted, punctuating each knee bend with a shake of both arms. He did it quickly, five times in row, as if under the spell of a strong spasmodic twitch. In the distance he heard the ball land.

Panting, he turned and looked at his brother, who looked back in stunned silence. As Jeff began walking toward the house in tears, his stomach sank. He knew his brother had seen it this time. He had seen his secret. He had seen his demon. He had seen the malfunctioning part of him that he had tried so hard to keep hidden. He felt diminished, damaged, flawed—no longer just the younger brother, but now the *imperfect* one as well.

He just knew things would never be the same between them.

Steve caught up with Jeff as he walked toward the screen porch.

"You OK?" he asked.

"I'm not feeling so good right now," Jeff said in a small voice. "I need to talk to Mom." Steve put his arm around his brother and walked him in to see their mother.

Inside, Patty Matovic had been watching out the kitchen window. "It was as if his entire body had been attached to a rope and it just went up and down, up and down, up and down," she recalled later. "It was like he was getting taller, then shorter, taller then shorter. It was mesmerizing."

She thought about a television program she had recently seen on Tourette Syndrome. She had noticed his nervous habits when he was younger. But everyone told her they were just phases that he would outgrow. Indeed, each habit seemed to be replaced by another. One day he would grunt, another he would clear his throat or hiss like a snake.

She tried to ignore them.

But she couldn't ignore this. It was the absolute worst thing she had ever seen him do. Immediately she suspected Jeff had Tourette's. And she knew her family was in big trouble.

"Mom," Jeff said, running into the kitchen. "Something happened outside. I don't know what it was. My body just acted all weird on me. Steve and I were playing catch and I just kind of . . . shook. I didn't mean to. It just happened."

They sat together on a padded red kitchen booth.

"I saw what happened," his mother said.

"You did?" Jeff said in a small voice.

"If we need to see a doctor about it, we will. But I don't want you to feel it's your fault. It's pretty clear that this was something you didn't want to do."

"OK," Jeff said, still confused.

"Why don't you go relax, watch TV, or play in your room," his mother said.

Her calm demeanor belied more serious concerns. Tourette's was a whole new world, both unfamiliar and frightening. And it was bound to change their lives.

She couldn't have known how much.

— ◆ —

WEEKS LATER JEFF waited in a neurologist's office in a three-story medical building in downtown Pittsburgh. His long legs dangled off the end of the examination table, keeping time like giant pendulums.

He stared straight ahead as he sat on a thin sheet of white paper waiting for a doctor he would have given anything not to see.

While he waited he imagined more dire possibilities. His shoulders slumped from worry.

"Sit up straight," his mother said, tugging at his shirt collar. The noodle-thin boy snapped his head around and pulled away from her touch. Her brown eyes softened.

"It's going to be OK, honey," she said, softly stroking the back of his closely cropped black hair. "We'll get through this together."

He closed his eyes and drew in a deep breath.

"Mom?" he said.

"Hmm?"

"Am I going to die?"

6

Dr. Dream Crusher

AS JEFF WAITED for the doctor he looked at a laminated poster of a brain tacked above a small sink. His wide eyes devoured every inch of the detailed illustration. It was so shiny, plump, and impressive. Its pink cerebellum and red frontal lobe seemed to glow with good health.

Now this was a brain, he thought. *The kind of brain everyone should have, the kind of brain that functioned properly without causing any kind of crazy problems.* Too bad it wasn't his brain. His brain was different. His brain was—bad!

He pictured it like an old mushroom, shriveled and shrunken in shades of black and gray. The longer he looked at the healthy brain on the wall, the madder he became.

"Look at me," it seemed to be saying. "I'm perfect. The perfect brain!"

He imagined it goading him in the singsong voice little kids used to tease each other.

You don't have what I've got. Nana-na-na-na-na!

His shoulders dropped. Not only was his brain not perfect, it probably was broken. Maybe he had brain cancer. What if he became paralyzed? Would he ever be able to go out and play with his friends again? The scary possibilities rolled around in his mind like a marble in a box.

"Mom?" Jeff said.

"Hmm?"

"Am I going to die?"

His mother turned to face him.

"*No*, honey. What would make you think that?"

"*Huh!*" Jeff said, forcing air from his mouth as his arm flew out from his side. "I don't know." His arm flew out several more times, followed by several hard leg swings that made him look like he was trying to kick a soccer ball.

"I'm sorry," he said.

"You don't have to apologize," his mother said, rubbing his cheek. The disturbing images of Tourette's from the television program she had watched raced through her mind. But she couldn't let Jeff see her concern. She took a breath and managed a smile.

"You're going to be fine," she said in a reassuring voice. "We just need to know a little more about what's going on so we can help you."

Jeff didn't want to be helped. He wanted to leave. He wanted to run, so fast and so far that no one could ever find him.

Then again, maybe his mom was right. Maybe he *was* going to be fine. He was a good student. He could think clearly and hold conversations. And he was very athletic. Maybe all he needed was to take a pill. Yeah. They had pills for everything!

He'd know soon enough. The doctor walked through the door.

TALL, THIN, AND serious, the middle-aged neurologist stared at his clipboard for what seemed like an eternity. Typically he saw elderly patients. Rarely did a child walk through the door.

Jeff's heart seemed to beat in his stomach and his throat at the same time. After walking across the small room the doctor sat down and jotted a few notes. It was only about ten seconds, but it was the longest ten seconds of Jeff's life.

Just tell me! Jeff thought. *Am I going to die? Live? How long do I have?*

The doctor began a standard examination, shining a light in Jeff's pupils and checking other vital signs while observing the variety of his tics. Jeff didn't like his new doctor. It was like being worked on by a mannequin. The brown-haired man in the white lab coat seemed callous, cold, and unemotional. He wore a neutral expression and worked almost robotically. Jeff scanned his face, looking for emotional reinforcement or reassurance. He wanted to hear that everything was going to be all right, that he could go on being a normal kid, that he wasn't going to die. All he got was the man's deep monotone telling him the bad news.

Jeff's mother knew what he was going to say. Still, she didn't want to hear it.

"I think this is Tourette Syndrome," he said. "But I'd like to schedule some tests to rule out other possibilities." Among other tests he scheduled a CAT scan to make sure Jeff didn't have a brain tumor.

It was the first time Jeff had heard the term *Tourette Syndrome*. It scared him. A *syndrome*? He didn't know what that was, but it didn't sound good. And what did the doctor mean he *thought* it was Tourette Syndrome? He didn't know? Jeff needed to know. He couldn't go home still wondering.

His mother needed more information too. "If this is Tourette's, are there medications that can help?"

"There's no one medication that always works," the doctor said. "It's trial and error. Dosages differ with each patient. But I'm afraid whatever we do, Jeff's tics will get a lot worse before they get better."

"What do you mean?" she asked, not sure she wanted to hear the answer.

"Jeff's going to most likely experience a lot of difficulty throughout his life," the doctor said. "He may not be able to finish high school or get the grades you'd want him to get."

Jeff felt a hollow, sinking feeling in his chest, as if the doctor's words had let all the air out of his body.

The doctor looked down to address Jeff directly. "This is most likely going to limit your ability to perform in any capacity," he said. "Seeing that you might need to go on medication, you're probably not going to be able to perform academically the way you want. I know this is a little hard for you to hear, but this is what I've dealt with in the past."

Jeff's mother asked questions with her eyes.

"Don't expect too much out of Jeff," the doctor said in response. "School is going to be difficult. He may not be able to graduate from high school. He may need to have provisions made for him. And don't get your hopes up for college. In the meantime let's continue to explore this. I have some more patients to meet with. I'll be in touch."

He wasn't a bad doctor, simply a formal one. Later Patty Matovic even worked for him for several months as an assistant office manager.

But to Jeff he wasn't a doctor but a dream crusher. Jeff wanted to play sports and go to college. He had plans, dreams. He wanted to help people. Could he do any of that now? It felt like his life was over before it had started.

In one way he was scared, but in another he was mad. That doctor didn't know anything about him. Who was he to limit him? What right did he have to snatch away his future?

He'd show him, the old jerk!

Jeff's mom had her own fears. How bad would her son's tics get, and how would he handle them? How would she? And what would it mean for her family?

7

Jumping Out of My Skin

I DIDN'T KNOW what was wrong with me until 1984. One day I went to a neurologist and he told me—just like that. I was twenty-six at the time, and had been married for four years.

Yes, having Tourette's was hard. But since I could hide the worst of it, it didn't stop me from falling in love.

I still remember how we met. In the fall of 1976, after graduating from Lincoln Southeast High School, I enrolled at the University of Nebraska. Like many of my friends I lived at home and commuted to the downtown campus. Most days I took the Arapahoe bus. The bus system in Lincoln was clean, well-run, and friendly—much like the city itself. When my classes were over, I'd wait for my bus at a shelter outside a Toyota dealership on the edge of campus.

It was there, on a cold and cloudy day in February 1977, that my life changed forever. I remember it as clearly as if it were playing on a Blu-ray disc. I was having a horrible day. I had lost my backpack with all my books, notes, and assignments in it, and failed a geology quiz I had forgotten about. To make myself feel better I bought some donuts on my way to the bus stop.

That's when I saw Susan sitting alone on the end of the bench. She was model pretty—slender and striking with blue eyes, porcelain skin, and a perfect figure. Her gently curled, shoulder-length strawberry blonde hair shone like a new penny.

I sat next to her, and—with great effort—managed to block my tics.

It started to rain.

"Perfect," I said, holding out a hand to feel the droplets blowing in on me under the smoky glass shelter. "Go ahead, rain on me! Everything else has happened to me today!"

I decided I was going to make something good happen. Right then.

I held out the bag. "Donut?" I asked her.

"Oh, no thanks," she said with a shy smile that lit up my heart like a blowtorch.

"Oh, come on," I cajoled, smiling, and turning on as much charm as I could muster. "Have one."

"No. I don't think so," she said, looking down shyly.

"Look," I said with a nothing-to-lose confidence, "something's got to go right today. Just have a donut. *One donut!* Would that kill you? I lost my backpack, I flunked a geology quiz, and now it's raining all over me. Make *one thing* go right today. Just let me give you a donut."

"OK," she relented, taking one from the bag.

I kept talking, and before long she began to smile at me in that way that seemed to say, *You're really weird, but you're kind of funny and sweet too.*

God, she was cute. I knew within a minute of seeing her I was going to get on any bus she got on, even if it took me twenty miles out of my way. I didn't care where I ended up—I wasn't about to let her get away. As it turned out, the bus she got on was my bus. She lived less than two miles from me. I remembered to get her full name—Susan Torpy—seconds before I got off.

That afternoon I called her for a date.

By August 1980 we were married.

Susan never seemed to mind my head movements. At least she never said so. Almost unbelievably, we never talked about them. I guess I covered well. To most people it just looked like I was vain, and liked to flip my longish brown hair to the right. Susan knew that I struggled; she was just too nice to say anything.

We were so happy. Young and in love, we didn't even know we were poor. After I finished up my political science degree in college, Susan worked three jobs as I studied to score high enough on the LSAT to earn a spot at the University of Nebraska School of Law.

At the time I thought I wanted to be a lawyer. I did fine in my classes but soon became disillusioned. There were too many things that bothered me, and I didn't want to stick it out just to wake up one day forty years later and decide I was unhappy.

There's nothing wrong with being a lawyer. It just wasn't for me. I remember one day having a discussion with my legal writing professor about the proper way to write a legal brief. He wanted me to use all those fancy fifty-cent lawyerin' terms that confuse regular people and keep lawyers rich because regular people need a lawyer to figure out what they mean. I wrote my legal brief in simple, unambiguous English.

He didn't like it. I didn't like him.

"If you want to write like that, go to journalism school," he said.

"OK," I said, "I will." And I did.

I loved journalism school. I had finally found my passion: words.

Through the help of my mentors Alfred "Bud" Pagel, Dick Streckfuss, and Jim Neal, I learned the craft quickly. I wrote articles for the J-school's paper and a regular column for the student newspaper, the *Daily Nebraskan*.

Before I knew it, Bud Pagel called me into his office and told me I should apply for an internship. Interviewers from top papers around the country would be visiting the school and interviewing students.

This was it—a way to get my foot in the door at a real newspaper! I signed up for numerous interviews with papers large and small. The two I was the most interested in were the two most prestigious internships: the *Miami Herald* and the *Wall Street Journal*.

I prepared for the *Wall Street Journal* interview first. I was so nervous as I waited to be called into the room, my head felt like it was strapped to an electric paint shaker.

Calm down, I told myself. *Breathe. Focus. Think about your answers.*

"Jim?" a middle-aged man with black hair and Wharton-Business-School glasses asked.

I walked into the interview room and sat down. The interview had barely gotten started when the no-nonsense interviewer noticed my odd head movements.

"Can you hide that?" he said, barely looking up from whatever he was reading.

"For a little while," I said. "If I try hard enough."

"I'd hide it if I were you."

Seriously? I thought. *That's your professional advice? And you call yourself a journalist? Aren't you the least bit curious about who I am, or why my head is shaking in the first place?*

I could have tried to turn it around. Made a joke. Used my charm. Or I could have told the greasy little weasel where he could stick his friendly recommendation. As the interview continued and he kept being an insensitive jerk, I decided he wasn't worth it. At this point I wouldn't have worked for him even if he offered me a job as the *Journal*'s Hawaii correspondent writing about hula girls for $100,000 a year.

My next interview was with Gene Miller and Mike Baxter, two Pulitzer Prize winners from the *Miami Herald*. The beginning of the interview, which took place in a small room at the University of Nebraska's school of journalism, went uneventfully. I told them about my tics, and they told me not to worry, that they wouldn't be a factor. How refreshing!

Gene Miller asked me to surprise them.

"Tell us something we wouldn't know," he said.

"All right," I said. "You and you are diaskeuasts."

"We're *what*?" a suddenly intrigued Miller asked, leaning forward in his seat.

"Diaskeuasts," I repeated confidently.

They looked at each other for a few seconds as I leaned back in my seat and smiled.

"What's a diaskeuast?" Miller asked.

I *had* them.

"I'll tell you the same thing my father always told me," I said. " 'Look it up.' I think there's a dictionary just outside the room." They left and returned a minute later with a fat *Webster's Third International Dictionary*. When they discovered what the word meant, they looked at each other and laughed. The word the two professional wordsmiths, the two Pulitzer Prize winners, the two men who would make a decision on my future, had never heard meant, simply, editor.

"That's great!" Miller said.

Later that month I was chosen for the internship. I went home and told Susan we were moving to Miami.

BEFORE WE LEFT for the Sunshine State, I went to a neurologist for the first time. But I might not have gone to him if it hadn't been for a friend named Chip Morris and his mother, Bernice.

One day Chip and I were sitting and talking between classes in Oldfather Hall on the campus of the University of Nebraska. I can't remember how we got on the subject of my head movements, but Chip knew I was struggling and wanted to help. He suggested I talk to his mother, a therapist.

Desperate for answers, I did. I met with Bernice Morris for several weeks before she looked at me and said, "Emotionally, there's nothing wrong with you. Have you ever considered that your movements might have a physical cause?"

A lightbulb turned on over my head.

"I never considered that," I said, pausing to wonder why. "My father always assumed my head shaking had a psychological or emotional trigger. That's all I've heard since I was small. I guess I just came to believe the same thing."

I drove home that day thinking in an entirely new way.

Physical?

It was an interesting theory. But what sort of physical ailment could cause this? Besides a little head shaking, I felt fine.

I put the thought out of my head. But several days later it came roaring back. I remember it like it was yesterday. I picked up a *Time* magazine and stared at a full-page advertisement bearing a large picture of William Shatner—Captain Kirk from *Star Trek*. The headline above his head read: DOES YOUR CHILD HAVE TOURETTE SYNDROME? DO YOU EVEN KNOW WHAT IT IS?

"No, Captain," I said playfully. "What is it?"

When I read the ad I shuddered. I read it again. Then I tore it out.

"Oh my God!" I said out loud. "This is *me*!"

A week later I sat in neurologist's office and listened as he changed my life.

"It's nothing much to worry about," he said, his voice trailing off. "It's a tic disorder. You've got a disorder called Tourette Syndrome."

"What?" I said, straining to hear. "What was the name?"

"Oh the name's not important," he said. "It's a tic disorder. You've got tics."

"*Dammit!*" I said, jumping from my seat and staring at him. "Don't tell me the name's not important. *Tell me the name!*"

"Tourette Syndrome," he said.

"Really?" I said. "You mean it's in the medical books? I haven't made it up? I'm not crazy?"

"You have tics," he said again.

"Stop saying that!" I said. "I have a name for it now. I have something to tell people. I can have a telethon for God's sake! I have Tourette Syndrome!"

I held my breath as my neurologist gave me a prescription for a powerful antipsychotic drug called Haldol that he said could lessen my head shaking, or maybe stop it altogether.

I ran to my car and shut the door. *Dad,* I thought as I turned the key, *it wasn't our fault. We didn't cause this.* I soon thought a lot of impossible things could come true.

It was almost too much to imagine. A new life? No more shakes? To be *normal?* I drove home to my apartment, dreaming of a life without a shaking head. At home I hugged Susan after showing her the pills. I knew she would love me whether they worked or not, but when I saw her face and the look in her eyes, I wanted them to work right then. I walked into the bathroom and took a pill. Three weeks passed with no reaction. My doctor increased my dosage. Soon after taking the stronger pill, I didn't want to shake my head.

I wanted to die.

The pills made me restless, many times worse than anything I had experienced from Tourette's.

I paced quickly around the apartment.

"What's wrong?" Susan asked.

I threw my hands up and continued to pace, changing directions like a tiger in a cage.

"You know that swirling energy that's usually in my head?" I said.

"Yes."

"Well it's in my chest and my stomach now. And it's like ten times stronger! I can't relax. I gotta move. I want to jump out of my skin."

Into the kitchen, onto the sofa, through the hallway, into the bathroom, out of the bathroom, I looked out the window, rolled on the floor, did jumping jacks and cooked two breakfasts I didn't want. Susan tried to hold me, but I broke free of her embrace. I wanted to move. I wanted to scream. I wanted to run.

That's it. I wanted to run. I went outside in my socks. Twelve degrees and snowing. I ran in a large circle in snow up to my calves. The cold and the exercise felt good. I didn't know it then, but I was experiencing a nasty side effect of the medication called akathesia, a condition of intense discomfort that—if bad enough—can lead to suicide or violence against others. I never wanted to hurt anybody. I just wanted the feeling to stop. I ran for twenty minutes as fast as I could until I had worn a smooth circular path in the apartment's unplowed parking lot. I came in exhausted. I don't know how I got to sleep that night, but in the morning I threw the Haldol away.

The doctor asked a lot of questions. "Do you remember the first time your body did something you didn't want it to do?" he asked. "A movement. A feeling. Something you couldn't control?"

My whole childhood came rushing back to me. I was born in 1958 in Philadelphia. The younger of two children, I had an older sister named Nancy. My parents were academics. My father, Jay, had a PhD in the history of religion. He both spoke and understood many languages, including Latin and German. His first real job was defining all the religion words for *Webster's Third International Dictionary*. He met my mother, who has a master's degree in religious education, at the University of Chicago Theological Seminary.

While they both attended that prestigious school, they were house parents for the Roby House, one of Frank Lloyd Wright's most famous architectural masterpieces. As smart as they were, they were not ready for what Tourette Syndrome was about to bring into their lives. But then, who could be?

I remembered the exact moment my head began to move. It was 1965, and I was seven years old. Every night Huntley and Brinkley would report the total dead in the Vietnam War over our black-and-white TV. I would root for our side, without even really knowing who or why we were fighting. At the same time my older sister, Nancy, was in love with this mop-haired group of musicians who called themselves the Beatles.

I was in the bathroom of my childhood house in Swarthmore, Pennsylvania. The shakes were small, imperceptible, more like subtle vibrations than the brutal brain shakers that would come later. I just kept watching my head, as if by looking at it I could somehow stop it, or understand it, when the truth was I really couldn't do either. So I stood there, transfixed, as the small but powerful impulses grew inside my head.

I didn't know what to think about the head vibrations, only that I didn't dare tell anybody about them. Although I didn't understand it then, I must have worried that if I talked about them that would somehow legitimize them, make them real, or make them worse. That scared me. Better to keep a lid on it as long as I could.

Of course I had Tourette's then. It was spreading, growing stronger, putting down its evil roots. I just didn't know it.

In the second grade I began shrieking like a teakettle. I didn't *want* to make the sound and tried everything to stop. I couldn't. I'd make the high-pitched sound repeatedly in the back of my throat when I became excited. I made the sound so much at school that I had to stay home from second grade for several months.

Throughout grade school I hid my tics as much as I could. I would shake or blink when I was alone, or when someone's back was turned. Of course there were times when someone would see me and say something. I used my sense of humor as a shield. I'd either make them laugh or quickly steer the conversation in another direction.

Most got the hint that I didn't want to talk about it.

Most.

Several times a classmate saw me sharply nodding my head forward in rapid succession and pointed and laughed. He said I needed "Nic-O-Nod," a medication he made up.

I didn't get any medications when I was a child. My parents did the best they could. But for some reason they were certain my problem was an emotional one. I saw several psychiatrists as a young boy. I played in dark-paneled rooms with darts and balls and board games, all designed to make me comfortable enough to open up to straightlaced strangers in dark suits. Most of the questions were of the "Are you having trouble in school?" or "Do you hate your parents?" variety. It didn't matter how many times I said no. They just kept asking.

Eventually my parents gave up on therapists and let me settle into my own pattern. They didn't have much choice. No one could tell them what was wrong with me.

That made my father crazy. Night after night he would call me into his room and try to find the problem. A smart man who was valedictorian of his high school class and went on to earn a PhD, he desperately wanted to fix me.

"What's bothering you, Jim?" he'd plead. And I would cry. I hated the pain in his eyes. I just wanted to stop so that he could stop.

I couldn't. So as a boy—and as an adult—I did the only thing I really knew how to do. Day by day, I simply survived.

8

My Search for Relief

SURVIVE? THERE ARE plenty of people who've known me for years who won't understand that. What does *he* have to survive?

But then they only know half of me—the part that's in excellent health. Truth is, I'm in excellent health and in agony at the same time. And for most of my life I've been pretty good at hiding the agony part.

It's a confusing way to live. A medical form once asked me to rate my health as excellent, good, fair, or poor. I honestly didn't know what to put. Susan suggested I split the difference and check "good." But that's not how I feel. I'm naturally positive, hopeful, and in many ways very healthy. I don't smoke, I don't drink, and I've never done drugs. I eat fresh fruits and vegetables, and exercise regularly by lifting weights, shooting baskets, riding my bike, and taking my cockapoo, Snickers, for five-mile walks. My favorite breakfast is a bowl of oatmeal with two tablespoons of milled flaxseed, banana slices, English walnuts, raisins, and skim milk. I take two baby aspirins a day, along with two multivitamin pills with special cholesterol-fighting ingredients, and six fish oil tablets. During winter I get fewer cold and flu viruses than my wife or kids. I never get headaches, I have an excellent sense of humor, and feel pretty happy most of the time.

On the other hand, when it comes to my Tourette's, I'm falling apart. I'm severely sleep deprived, have a constant pain in my neck and my brain, and sometimes feel dizzy or worry that one day I'm just going to fall down or die.

But then I'll have a day where I am inexplicably happy. I can't help it. That's just how I am. Hence my dilemma. Am I the sickest healthy person you'll ever meet, or the healthiest sick person? I'm both. And that's why it's so hard for anyone to understand me.

As my age increased, so did my pain and my determination to find relief.

Many people have asked me why I never drank or took drugs to dull the pain. The answer is simple. I'm not an idiot. Self-medicating is not dealing with your pain, it's masking it. Plus drugs are illegal, and alcohol tastes like tooth medicine. Over the years my search for legal relief has involved many things, including:

Pillows

While I don't know the reason, sometime in my midforties sleeping in a bed grew increasingly uncomfortable. I began sleeping on the living room floor. Initially I blamed it on my pillow. Maybe after years of trauma, I thought, my neck needed different support.

I bought new pillows in stores and online. I bought them from shopping channels and late-night infomercials. I bought down pillows, memory foam pillows, pillows recommended by celebrities, and pillows that supposedly changed people's lives.

Deep down I knew they wouldn't work. But when you're desperate, you cling to hope like a life preserver. Susan turned the channel if she saw a pillow ad. She knew I'd buy it. She also knew it wouldn't work. Reluctantly, I came to believe her. It wasn't all bad, though. I had a great time with the pillows. One of my happiest memories is building a pillow wall with my daughter. One day when Allison was seven I stacked pillows in our bedroom doorway until they formed a giant wall. Then I invited Allie to run through them. For years this was our favorite game. After picking out her favorite pillows, she would take several steps into the hallway and get ready to run through the giant wall.

"Are you ready?" I'd ask. She'd smile and nod her head excitedly.

"One, two, three . . . GO!"

Allie would run as fast as she could, her blonde hair bobbing behind her, and crash through the wall like a superhero. She'd tumble into our bedroom and giggle until her face was red.

"Again!" she'd shout. And I didn't care how much pain I was in. I would build that pillow wall as many times as she wanted. I'll never forget the first time we did it.

"I love you, Daddy!" she said afterward, running up to me. A tear ran down my face as my little girl hugged me around my aching neck.

"I love you too, princess," I said.

When we were through she skipped away the happiest girl in the world. And at that moment I didn't care how much I spent on those pillows. The look in her eyes was worth every penny.

Mattresses

When pillows did not bring me relief, I settled on a new villain: our mattress. Susan and I had slept on same one for twenty years. After buying a new king-size, I slept pain-free for the first time in years. I knew it. I wasn't getting worse. It was just the mattress!

Except it wasn't. The second night I tossed and turned. By the end of the week I was sleeping on the floor.

Still, I was convinced the mattress was the problem.

One day I thought I found the answer in a local furniture store. As my wife shopped for new bedroom furniture for Allie, I stretched out on an adjustable bed. I fell asleep raising and lowering my head and my legs, then woke up to the sound of a salesman.

"Comfortable model, isn't it?" he said.

"Uh, sure is," I said, wiping my mouth as I sat up, hoping I hadn't drooled on the pillow.

"Relax," he said. "That's what it's there for. Just let me know if I can help you take one home."

He handed me his card and left. I got up to check the price.

Six *thousand* dollars!

My heart sank, but I couldn't stop thinking about it. At work I gushed about the bed to my oldest friend at the paper, the *Star*'s national correspondent, Rick Montgomery. Rick had a theory. The up-and-down bed worked because instead of fighting my tics, I was finally giving them what they wanted—movement.

Maybe he was right. But $6,000?

After some research I bought one online for less than $5,000. I was excited when it arrived. But over the next week I tried to make it work like the one in the store, *but could* never repeat the feeling. Back it went.

Massages and Hot Tubs

Massages help me more than anything. Problem is, they're expensive, and the benefit lasts only several hours. For years I had a massage every week. The treatments were partially paid for by insurance. As great as they felt, the long-term cost—in both money and time—was still too much. I worked out a compromise with my insurance company. I would stop getting massages if they would pay for half the cost of a whirlpool. After many meetings they agreed, and I put the spa in my basement. For years it has been one of my most reliable forms of relief.

Mötley Crüe

When nothing else helps and I absolutely cannot stand the pain, I can always use my secret weapon to distract me from the pain for a few minutes. I sit at my computer, put on my headphones, and listen to rock songs at ear-splitting levels. Over the years many songs have helped me. My current favorite is "Kickstart My Heart" by Mötley Crüe. I listen to it over and over. I can't explain why it helps. There's just something about the driving rock beat—the tone and the tempo throbbing through my Sennheiser headphones straight into my brain—that takes away my pain.

It's wonderful! I also think there's something marvelously appropriate about the name of the album the song comes from: *Dr. Feelgood.*

Couldn't have said it better myself.

Aquamassage

During a family vacation, as we were strolling around Branson Landing on the Missouri waterfront, we walked past a booth featuring an Aquamassage machine. The large contraption was about ten feet long, featured a bright blue acrylic top, and opened like a coffin. *Aquamassage?* I wondered. I didn't want to get wet.

Actually, the operator said, since the water jets would massage me through a thin plastic barrier, I wouldn't—and I could keep my clothes on.

"Do it, Daddy!" Allison said.

It wasn't expensive. And I *was* hurting.

Fine. I rolled in on my stomach and put my face in the soft, supportive, open pad—the same kind used by massage therapists. Then, using a controller, the operator slowly closed the lid and fired her up.

The great beast roared to life and began to fire powerful water jets at me. The water was warm. It started on my feet, moved up my legs, onto my back, and up to my neck. Then it began to pulsate, slow at first, then incredibly fast and powerful. I had a button to stop the movement wherever I wanted.

I stopped it on my neck—and left it there.

Oh . . . My . . . God!

I had never felt anything as relaxing. The power and warmth of the pulsating jets stunned my Tourette's and obliterated the pain and tightness in my neck. After ten minutes, when my session was over, the operator almost had to wake me up. Incredibly, I was pain free. Driving back to our room, I turned to my family—and actually got mad.

"*This* is how you feel?" I asked. "All the time?"

My poor wife didn't know what to say.

"THIS IS HOW YOU FEEL?" I said. "No pain at all? Completely relaxed? LIKE THIS?"

It suddenly dawned on me. "Why the hell should I do *anything* for you when you feel like this all the time? *You* go to work full-time! *You* rake the leaves and mow the lawn!" I stared straight ahead with pursed lips and angry eyes as the slightest bit of pain slowly began to creep back into the side of my neck.

I later apologized. It's just that when you live with pain every second it's hard to get a glimpse of what it would be like to live without it—especially when you know it's not going to last. That's when I had a crazy thought.

Maybe it *could* last? What if I bought an Aquamassage machine for my house?

When I got home I got online and started pricing a machine. Turns out they only cost . . . *thirty thousand dollars*?

I couldn't give up. I wouldn't! I found a used one online for $6,500. I had it shipped to my home and put in my basement. The first week it brought relief for a half a day or more. But the more I used it, the more my Tourette's adapted to it. I can't explain it, but Tourette's is a chameleon. After something gives me relief, my tics often "fight back" as if they know I'm trying to reduce them.

The machine still relieved my pain, but the relief dropped to an hour. It was still worth it. And it continued to help me for months afterward—until it started to leak.

I got bad news from the company. Kansas City had no Aquamassage repairmen. I would have to fix it myself. I ordered a new moisture seal from the company and, with a little coaching from the service techs, managed to disassemble it and install the new seal. The challenge: getting it back together.

Not easy. The machine sat broken in my basement for more than a year. Finally, I called several local spa and pool companies. None had heard of an Aquamassage. And only one—Pool & Patio—had someone willing to take a shot at fixing it. The next day a technician named Troy Falder came to my house. I didn't think he'd be able to fix it, but to my surprise, he did. In less than an hour he had it reassembled and working!

I couldn't believe it! I was so happy I gave him a $200 tip.

So, yes, the machine is working again. And it helps. Unfortunately, the more I use it, the more my Tourette's adapts to it. The pain relief now is pretty much limited to when I am in the machine.

Even More Relief

The pillows, mattresses, massages, whirlpool, and Aquamassage are only a small fraction of the things I've done to get relief. I've also gone to doctors, seen therapists, and bought massagers, head scratchers, neck squeezers, roller balls, and a gravity inversion table. I've had acupuncture and practiced tai chi and Qui Gong meditation. Occasionally I wear a towel around my shoulder to cushion the blow of my shakes, and stretch strong elastic workout bands around my neck to ease the pain. I've taken Haldol, Klonopin, Catapress, Pimozide, Zanaflex, Valium, Vicodin, high doses of fish oil, and used every over-the-counter pain-relieving tablet or rub on the market.

Special diets? Check.

Allergy shots. Yup.

Watching TV helps, but I can't watch twenty-four hours a day. Listening to loud music helps, but if I listen as loudly as I want I'll be deaf by sixty. I listen to the Rolling Stones sing "19th Nervous Breakdown" and think, *Yeah, that's about right.*

After trying almost everything, I figured there wasn't anything left to try.

I was wrong.

One day I discovered a product I never knew existed: a thigh-sized blood pressure cuff. Then it hit me. That might feel amazing on my head! It could equalize pressure, even take away pain. And while a regular cuff wouldn't fit my head, a thigh-sized one certainly would. Excited, I bought one and inflated one around my head. The pressure eliminated my pain. The problem: it covered my eyes and smashed my nose.

I called several companies to ask them if they could make a headband-shaped inflation device. One by one they told me they didn't do such things. Finally, one company said it would—for $4,000.

Finally I called Sealtech in Athens, Tennessee, and talked to a man named James Winder.

Please, Lord, I prayed. *Let him understand my pain.*

James had a Southern accent, a kind voice, and a respectful way about him. And to my surprise he didn't tell me custom-making a device was impossible, or shoo me off like all the others.

"Listen," I said. "I know companies don't usually work like this. It's not your job to care about the needs of one person."

"Sometimes it is," he said. "We're all our brother's keeper."

It was one of the kindest things anyone ever said to me. James said he'd check with his engineers. When he called back, shortly before Christmas, he told me the good news.

"I'm going to do something for you," he said, describing an inflatable headband his company could make that sounded like the answer to my prayers.

He then apologized.

"I wanted to be able to give this to you for free," he said. "Would . . . $200 be too much?

Two hundred dollars? I could have hugged him through the phone. It was a Christmas miracle!

It was on that day that James Winder became one of my personal heroes, and Sealtech one of my favorite companies. The product arrived several weeks before Christmas. When I put it on my head and pumped it up, it temporarily relieved the pressure in my head. That night I said a prayer of thanks for James and his coworkers.

Some say corporations are evil. That's not what I found at Sealtech—just decent people who cared enough to help someone they'd never met. These are people who should be proud to look themselves in the mirror at night. They didn't take away my tics, but they did make them easier to endure. And for that I will never be able to say thank you enough.

It isn't perfect, though. Nothing ever is with Tourette Syndrome.

I still have pain and stress. I still have frustration and sadness. And there are days that are so hard, so horrible, so filled with desperation and loneliness that sometimes I just feel like giving up.

9

I'd Rather Have Cancer

THIS MIGHT SOUND crazy, but some days I'd rather have cancer than Tourette Syndrome. I'm not talking about the really horrible kind that destroys lives and tears families apart; I mean the kind doctors have a shot at curing.

I don't mean to be insensitive. I have friends with cancer. I've seen people *die* from cancer. So why make that statement?

I'm just jealous of the attention and understanding. People don't understand the suffering involved with serious, lifelong Tourette Syndrome. Not even my own family understands.

Not really.

But I hear you. *You don't know the first thing about how frightening cancer is! And why would you ever want to trade Tourette's for cancer? Tourette's is not fatal!*

True. But then, some days, that's the problem. It gets awfully lonely in this body. I've endured the tics, the pain, and the embarrassment of Tourette's for half a century. If I want any understanding at all, I have to *tell* people how much I'm suffering, which isn't cool.

When you have cancer, everyone understands immediately that you're *really sick*. You might have to have radiation or chemotherapy. Your hair might fall out. You might gain weight, lose weight, or your personality might change. Then there's the little fact that your condition may just *kill* you. Who doesn't understand that?

And so you get immediate attention. People with Oh-my-God faces come to talk to you. They bring food to your house and take up collections, because—for God's sake—*you've got cancer*!

Nobody's ever done that for me because I just have something that makes my head move, and occasionally I look like I'm in some pain.

When you have cancer there are so many people rallying to your side, telling you how strong you are. They pray for you and remind you that you're not alone. *I've seen it.* They come to your desk and to your house, wear pink ribbons, hold your hand and give you hugs. They touch your shoulder and say, "Whatever I can do, just let me know."

There are cancer hospitals, cancer centers, and cancer support groups. There are cancer blogs, cancer message boards, and countless cancer fund-raising runs. There are even commercials for cancer hospitals that remind you that *there is hope for you*, that *you can beat this*, because there are entire teams of talented and compassionate cancer specialists fighting just for you.

Nobody's fighting for me. Not really.

The American Cancer Society has been around for one hundred years and has raised billions of dollars. By comparison, the far smaller Tourette Syndrome Association may as well be invisible. But if I had cancer? I just might have a fighting chance for the disease to go into remission, or to whip it entirely. Then look at me. *I beat cancer!*

"I can't believe how brave you are," people would tell me. "You're a cancer survivor!"

I hate to be petty, but *I'm* a survivor as well. I've survived *fifty years* of Tourette Syndrome. No one realizes how hard it has been. There's no medicine to stop my pain because I'm causing it myself. And since I've damaged the vertebrae in my neck, many days are pure torture. They shoot horses that have less pain.

And almost *nobody* says anything to me.

Am I whining? Sure I am. But after fifty years, I've earned the right.

Some tell me I'm nuts for preferring cancer to Tourette's. They tell me I must be kidding. I'm not. After suffering with painful and embarrassing tics through the better part of six decades, I am serious when I say there is something attractive about even a terminal cancer diagnosis. Sure, it would be scary. But at least in many cases it would be all or nothing. Either you beat it and it's over, or it kills you and it's over.

Even if it goes away and comes back, at least the suffering would have stopped for a little while. My suffering *never* stops. Too many days I feel utterly alone and helpless. I feel adrift, abandoned, a sick nobody, a forgotten orphan of pain.

With serious Tourette's there's no rest. There's no cure. There's just you and your willpower. How much can you take? Tourette's isn't a tumor you can cut out or something that bends easily to the will of pharmaceuticals. The evil is not only inside of you, it *is* you. It's part of you like your thoughts are part of you. It hurts you, controls you, embarrasses you. But the absolute worst thing Tourette's does is *destroy your sense of hope.*

No—I don't *really* want cancer. I just want the support it brings. Maybe if I had cancer people would squeeze my hand and tell me how strong I am. Maybe I wouldn't feel like I had to chop off my arm so they could see my pain. That's why if I could swap my Tourette's for cancer, I'd do it before the end of this sentence.

If you have cancer, please know I am not trying to marginalize your experience. I will never know the fear or the pain that you have faced. But then, you will never know the fear or the pain that I've faced either. Despite the fact that some people *do* understand my condition, every year there has been at least one person who has reminded me to keep it in perspective. It could be worse, they tell me. I could have— terminal cancer.

Ah, the trump card. No, Tourette's isn't going to kill me. I can live with it, work with it, and play with it. *Hell, I'm lucky!*

Then tell me this: why don't I feel lucky?

10

I Know How to Kill My Tourette's

ONE STEP. ONE step off the roof and it would all be over.

In the summer of 2003, as a warm breeze buffeted my short-sleeved black shirt like a flag, I stood at the edge of the rock-covered roof of my mother's retirement complex in Lincoln, Nebraska, and pondered the fragility of life. I kicked a pebble and watched it tumble off the front of the off-white building and drop to the ground, six stories straight down. I watched as it bounced off a concrete walkway, then nestled in the grass.

Ow! I clamped both hands around the back of my head, and closed my eyes as electric pain flashed through the back of my neck and settled in the base of my brain. And for a moment—one awful, wonderful moment—I imagined falling from that building, sailing headfirst through the wind toward that very walkway, eyes closed, finally free!

I managed a crooked smile. If my head hit the concrete from that distance it would explode like an overripe cantaloupe.

What would you do then, Satan? I asked, talking to my Tourette's. *'Cause that would be it for you!*

No more pain. No more torture. No more smiling through the agony or pretending to be all right. No more stupid comments or funny looks. No more enduring the unendurable, or explaining the unexplainable.

And no more being alone.

Yeah. I knew how to kill my Tourette's.

One step. One swan dive. One final *fucking* sayonara.

I stared across O Street, the busiest street in the city, to the bustling Westfield Shopping Mall. I looked at the hundreds of cars and wondered if any of the people in them could see me standing at the edge of the roof. I wondered how they'd feel if they suddenly saw me hurtle to the ground like a lawn dart.

I looked up, then looked down. I sighed and swallowed hard. And then I took one large step . . . back from the edge.

I'd never really do it. But I won't deny that there is a certain power—and freedom—in knowing that I could.

Don't screw with me, Satan, 'cause I'll put you in the ground! Just remember who's boss.

I walked back to the middle of the roof, where I sat with my back against a large wooden air-conditioning enclosure. I played with the rocks and tried to find a pretty one to keep. The sun felt good on my face as I thought about my time at the edge.

I had found the roof years ago while exploring. I went there to be alone. And for one reason or another, I always wound up at the edge. The people looked so small and insignificant from that height. And, sometimes, that's how I felt.

It was easy to feel sorry for myself up there. No one understood me. My kids didn't appreciate me. And after twenty-five years my wife said she loved me, but I knew it wasn't the same. *I* wasn't the same. I wasn't as fun-loving—not like I used to be—and I knew she had grown tired of hearing of my pain.

Who could blame her? Or the kids?

But then, what was the point of all this suffering again? You think about such things at the edge of a roof.

Suicide is many things to many people. For some it's the ultimate middle finger to an unfair world. For others it's the final end to intractable pain. For me, if I ever got to that point, it would be both those things. But mostly it would be a way of asking, "Now do you understand how much I was hurting?"

No. I'd never do it. But tell me, how many years of pain I am supposed to endure before I'm allowed to say, "I just can't stand this anymore!"

For Jeff, that number was thirty-one.

11

Butter and Salt on Your Neurons?

University Hospitals, Cleveland, Ohio. February 9, 2004.

Lying awake on an extra-long surgical table, Jeff stared into a bank of white-hot lights in an operating room so large you could kick a football in it. Jeff had had surgeries before—on a hand, several on his knees, and also for a hernia and his appendix. But he had never seen an operating room as enormous, elaborate, or high-tech. A wall of monitors faced the operating table, and two dozen finely detailed pictures of his brain hung around the room.

For months, a team laid the groundwork for the operation. Jeff's neurosurgeon identified a "target" deep inside Jeff's thalamus, the portion of the brain involved in controlling movement. The neurologic team mapped out regions of his brain using magnetic resonance imaging scans and 3-D computer images to determine exactly where the electrode should be placed, and the safest and most direct way to reach it.

Precision was paramount. If they missed the target by even a couple of millimeters the operation could fail. Furthermore, the surgeon would have to rely on his detailed knowledge of anatomy to reduce the risk of having the electrode act as a small spear through blood vessels or sensitive structures.

It was almost time to enter Jeff's brain. The trajectory had been chosen, the electrode driver had been mounted on the stereotactic frame holding Jeff's head still, and the angles and distances had been adjusted from the "magic numbers" obtained from the computer. All his surgeon had to do now was finish drilling the holes and remove the dura mater, the tough layer between the skull and the brain.

The high-pitched whine of the drill chewing through his skull seemed like it would never stop. But then—

"We're in," his surgeon said.

Jeff had known for months that they were going to drill holes in his head. Now that they had, it was almost too much to process. He tried to cover his nervousness with humor. "What do you mean you're in?" he asked. "You're in my *brain*? Can I look? What's in there? Probably not much, right?"

He slapped his right thigh. "Boy, talk about your invasion of privacy."

His surgeon couldn't help but smile.

"Hey, Doc," Jeff said playfully. "That was a Craftsman drill, wasn't it?"

"Only the best for you, Jeff."

As electronic devices beeped and hummed like a medical symphony, his esteemed doctor bent over the back of Jeff's head. He spoke in a calm and measured voice as comforting as an old sweater.

"Just want you to know we are going to get started," he said. "We're going to do the right side first."

The eight-hour operation was slow and tedious. Jeff's two doctors— his neurosurgeon and his neurologist—were joined by an electroneurodiagnostic technologist. Carefully, she passed a rigid microrecording electrode as thin as a human hair through Jeff's brain. The incredible sensitivity of the microrecording electrode allowed her to listen to one cell firing at a time. For doctors, who knew how to interpret the brain's Morse code, it was like a medical road map to Jeff's brain.

Jeff couldn't see what his doctors were doing, but he could hear it. It sounded like popcorn popping in a microwave. Some of the pops came slowly, others more quickly.

"What's that sound?" he asked his neurologist, who now had joined his colleague.

"Your neurons talking to each other," said his neurologist.

"You mean . . . I'm listening to my brain talk to itself?" Jeff said.

"That's right."

Jeff listened to the neurochemical symphony, wondering what his brain was saying. That he could even hear it was a miracle of modern science. It was hard to feel anything less than amazed as he realized he was thinking about the surgery with the same malfunctioning brain that doctors were trying to fix.

It was all so surreal. What must it look like in there? And how could they be *sure* about what they were doing?

Just relax and let them do their jobs, he thought.

Outside, in a small room, family and friends prayed and waited for news from the operating room. Jeff's father believed they would know immediately if the operation had been successful—if it was going to stop Jeff's tics.

That wasn't the case. Surgeons would leave uncapped wires sticking out of Jeff's skull. Then they'd have to do another surgery to implant battery packs in his pectoral muscles. Later still they'd have to adjust the frequency of his stimulators.

It would be a month before they knew if the operation had worked. Jeff hadn't told his parents much about the surgery other than his sincere belief that it would work. He hadn't told them about the possible complications. And he certainly hadn't told them that the next time deep brain stimulation worked on someone with Tourette Syndrome would be the first time. He didn't tell them because he didn't want them to worry—or worse, talk him out of it.

When the doctors came out of the surgery, Jeff's father anxiously peppered them with questions.

"It went very well," Jeff's neurosurgeon said. "Fantastic."

"So it *worked?*" Jeff's father asked.

"Well, we're not sure if it worked yet," the doctor said.

Jim Matovic's face fell as he found out his son would need more surgery on February 20 to implant batteries in his chest, and then come back a third time in March to see if everything worked. Deeply disappointed, he turned and walked away, needing to be by himself. The next month would be the longest of his life.

12

"I Need You to Cover Oprah"

IT WAS A Monday in early March 2004, and I was just getting to work a little after 9:00 AM.

I felt like a bag of wet cement. Sleep deprivation will do that to you.

After walking a block from the parking lot, up two flights, and across the width of the *Kansas City Star* building, the long hallway that led to the features department seemed even longer. Shambling more than walking, I trudged dead-eyed and silent past chipper colleagues who offered their morning greetings. I didn't dare look at them. I had to focus to keep Satan in his box.

Pain shot up the back of my neck. I wanted to scream.

I had to work.

If anyone can understand the agony that caused Jeff Matovic to beg doctors to bore into his brain, it's me. As a feature writer for the *Kansas City Star* for more than a quarter century, understanding people is a part of my job. And as someone who has struggled with Tourette's for the better part of fifty years, agony is a part of my life.

As a seven-year-old I ran through the streets of Swarthmore, Pennsylvania, shrieking like a teakettle. When I outgrew that, I began blinking and sniffing. By age ten I started nodding my head forward with quick, sharp snaps. I looked like a chicken buck-bucking its way around the henhouse. By the time I reached high school my head tic changed directions, moving left then whipping hard back to the right as if I were flipping my long brown bangs to one side. At the same time my head tic also changed in strength, adding a frightening violence to its sideways snap. I often shook my head so hard I could hear the thud my brain made when it slammed into the inside of my skull. Sure it hurt.

But it was never the pain that caused me the worst problems—at least at that point in my life. The worst thing about shaking your head in public is the way people respond to you. Some laugh. Others point. A few make comments. Everybody notices. And it hurts.

But what are you going to do? After you're all cried out you just try to find the humor in it. One time I shook my head so hard at a University of Kansas football game that my reading glasses flew off and landed in a drunk woman's beer. Try having *that* conversation.

Thankfully, my head tics had been relatively tame. Many others with Tourette's have had it so much worse. But in the winter of 2004 my embarrassing head tics became far more serious. Almost overnight they seemed to increase in frequency, intensity, and variety. The biggest changes were internal; new anxieties and tensions, the excruciating way I had to wrench my neck, and a handful of other painful movements that defy easy description. Overnight, it seemed, it became intolerable to sleep in a bed, something I had enjoyed for more than four decades. It didn't make sense that it was my Tourette's. It *had* to be the bed.

In the next two years I bought four king-sized mattresses that I also couldn't sleep in before giving up and defaulting to the living room floor. On my worst days I wasn't comfortable anywhere. I wanted to jump out of my skin and run away from a body that no longer seemed to want me in it. I ignored the pain. I smiled and made jokes. But inside I grew tired of the fight.

One day at work it became too much. Keith Robison, a lanky editor with a big heart and politically incorrect wisecrack for every occasion, picked up on my discomfort.

"Y'OK?" he asked in a big voice.

"I don't know," I responded in a small one.

He opened his arms and flashed a familiar smirk.

"Man hug?" he said.

I didn't want to smile, but I did anyway as I held up my hand to the big goofball as if to say, "I'm good."

I wasn't. I had two stories to write and no energy to write them.

"Good morning!" chirped Kady McMaster, an editor and longtime friend. "And how is Mr. Jim today?"

Mr. Jim felt like crap. I looked at my happily smiling coworker for a moment as I pondered what to say that wouldn't be a lie but would still uphold the social convention of the moment.

"I'm here," I said, grinning through sharp pains in my neck that were quickly joined by several waves of dizziness.

"Are you sleeping any better?" Kady asked with hopeful eyes.

God, how I wanted to say yes. How fun would *that* have been?

"Slept like a baby last night," I'd say. "I feel wonderful!"

But I didn't want to lie. And I didn't want to tell the truth. I hesitated, as my sleep-deprived brain searched for words.

"No?" Kady said.

"Not really," I said, almost apologetically.

As I reached my corner desk and plopped in my chair—a gray, coffee-stained, high-backed model that creaked when I sat down—I closed my eyes and fought back against the increasing tension. My neck moved like a rusty door hinge, and the muscles contracted as if being squeezed in a vise. Short of going into the fetal position, I couldn't find a comfortable place for my head.

A friend came over to talk. Without explanation, I excused myself and walked to the bathroom. I didn't need to go; I just needed to be alone. Sitting in the stall, I sighed as my head started to spin after several sharp shakes gave me one of my daily mini-concussions.

"Leave me alone," I moaned quietly, as I leaned my head on a plastic toilet paper dispenser and cried until tears fell on my black oxfords. I had been through hard times before. You don't survive as long as I have without being tough. But I'm not a machine. For the first time I began to wonder how long I could keep going before I cracked, fainted, quit, or died.

After twenty minutes I got up and looked at myself in the mirror. I chided myself for how weak I had grown. In my head I heard my father's voice.

"Hold your head high," he'd say. "We don't need their pity. We're Fussells! We're better than that." Except I wasn't. I was tired and I hurt. And I desperately wanted to tell someone how poorly I was feeling. I splashed cold water on my face, slapped my cheek, and pounded my forehead three times with a closed fist.

"Come on, Jim," I said.

The building pressure in my head pushed on the inside of my skull and squeezed my brain until it left its signature cold, empty pain. My head felt like it was going to explode.

At that moment I thought of my friend and coworker John Martellaro. He told me a story once about a politician he covered in Bucks County, Pennsylvania, who shocked everyone by pulling out a gun during a press conference and blowing off his head live on local television.

The pain increased inside my head again, pulsing like a flashing red light at an intersection. I moved my neck. It felt like I had pinched a nerve. *Fuck!*

I winced and thought about that guy from Pennsylvania. I checked to see if anyone else was in the bathroom, even stooping to look under the stalls. Then I took my index finger and thumb and made a gun, and jammed it into the back of my mouth, pointing up toward my brain. I imagined cold, hard steel against my teeth as I bit down while fingering the trigger.

It could be over just like that, I thought snapping my finger.

Blam!

Over!

Blam!

Done.

Blam!

Fuck you!

Just then I heard the bathroom door opening. I hurriedly took my finger out of my mouth and wiped it on the front of my shirt.

"Mr. Fussell," said Tim Engle, a friend from features who often greeted colleagues with an exaggerated formality.

"Mr. Engle," I said in return. He headed for the urinal; my gaze returned to the mirror.

Three hours' sleep again. I looked haggard and drawn. My eye bags had eye bags.

What had happened to me? When I was in my twenties and thirties my tics were easier to handle. I was bulletproof then—strong, fast, and flexible. I slept like Rip Van Winkle and had so much energy I could play thirty-six holes of golf, three sets of tennis, and a couple games of tackle football without feeling tired. My metabolism was so high I could eat as much as I wanted without gaining an ounce. At five feet ten, 155 pounds, I dunked volleyballs and leapt over parking meters with a forty-inch vertical leap. I was going strong at thirty-five and felt fine at forty. But when I reached forty-five my body began to break down. I felt aches and pains I never felt before. I couldn't sleep, and I had to eat twice as much just to keep up my strength. I ate so much my weight shot up to 215 pounds, twenty-five pounds heavier than I'd like. Before I knew it I had become exhausted, hurt, old, and fat. Worse, I was starting to have memory problems. As I sat looking at my computer login screen, I couldn't remember my password. Was it just the toll of middle age, or had all the shaking finally damaged my brain?

Great! I thought as I stared at the screen. *What now?*

"Think," I whispered under my breath. "Think. Think." It was like urging a car with a temperamental transmission, "Go."

I sat in silence, not moving, trying to remember my password, holding my head with my right hand to keep it steady. When the Tourette's was this bad I didn't make a sound. It must have been a relief to members of the nearby copy desk. In past years I had been such a loudmouth they occasionally had to tell me to pipe down. But when the tics are at their worst, I don't talk at all. If I'm in intense pain I might gasp or whimper, or pound on my desk with a closed fist. But I won't talk unless I have to. If I don't focus I'll hurt myself with head shakes so powerful they could knock me down—or knock me out.

After remembering I had written my password down, I logged on and leaned back in my chair. Then, wham! My powerful neck turned my head softly to the left, then snapped it hard back to the right. It felt like I'd been tagged by Mike Tyson. I slumped in my chair and started to moan as the pain increased. Desperate to end the assault, I distracted myself by walking around the newsroom. But glancing around just made me mad. I looked at my coworkers, happily typing away or talking on the phone with remarkably still heads. And for a moment I hated them. They made it look so easy. They just came in and started working. Just like that. What did they ever do to deserve such an advantage?

I closed my eyes as the tension closed around me like a vise. I cried softly as I tried to beat it back. I wanted to go home. I wanted to soak in a bath until I wrinkled like a shar-pei. I wanted to eat. I wanted to get on my computer and play music at ear-splitting decibels.

I couldn't think. It was never this bad. I started to panic. Was this what my life had become?

I sat down in a chair next to my editor, Sharon Hoffmann. I began to explain how I felt and that I was sorry, but I just couldn't finish a story she was expecting that day. Before I knew it, everything just overwhelmed me. I tried to stay strong. I tried to stay professional. It was no use. I was too tired. As I talked about what was wrong, I began to cry—and I just couldn't stop.

"Why don't you just go home," Sharon said. "It'll be all right."

"I'd love to," I said, blinking back the tears. "I can't. Don't you see? If I go home now it will have beaten me. And I'll be *damned* if I'm gonna let this thing beat me!"

I didn't look at anyone as I walked back to my desk. I put on my headphones and played "Behind Blue Eyes" by the Who. That song always made me feel better.

Roger Daltrey sang about how I felt.

No one knows what it's like

To be the bad man . . .

To be the sad man . . .

Behind blue eyes.

I closed my blue eyes as I sang along in my mind, letting the music wash over me. Music had always been able to do things that medicine couldn't. Before the song ended, my phone rang. I took off the headphones and stretched until my vertebrae popped.

"No pain," I whispered to myself under my breath. "No pain."

"The *Kansas City Star*," I said. "This is Jim Fussell speaking. May I help you?"

THE NEXT DAY was almost as hard, as was the day after that. My tics had changed, and like it or not, I would just have to learn to live with the increasing pain. Later that week I finished the other stories I was working on, making deadline with each one. The next time I talked to Sharon she had a new assignment for me.

"I need you to cover Oprah Winfrey" she said.

I blinked twice and furrowed my brow. *Oprah?*

Oprah, it seemed, was coming to Kansas City with a traveling beauty and empowerment workshop for women called Hi Gorgeous. The sold-out extravaganza created a buzz the likes of which I hadn't seen in the city for years. Some reports had tickets for the event going on eBay for more than $1,000. And as a feature writer for the *Star*, I was there to cover it. And her.

By all rights I shouldn't have gotten the assignment. That should have gone to my friend and colleague Lisa Gutierrez. Lisa, a terrific writer, was one of the biggest Oprah fans in the office. But she also was a professional who already was committed to another story she simply couldn't postpone.

"So could *you* do it?" Sharon said, folding her hands into a pretty-please posture.

Oprah? I thought. *What do I know about Oprah?* Then again, what did I know about anything I wrote about before I started?

"For you, anything," I said.

Sharon flapped her arms and gave me her goody-goody smile.

"All right, don't get too excited," I said.

All I knew about Oprah were the same things everybody knew. She was the queen of daytime, a billionaire power broker and star maker, and her most fanatical followers loved her with a breathless passion. I filled in the rest with my research and decided to write a story about her amazing popularity, her loyal followers, and—of course—that she and her crew were coming to Kansas City.

Naturally, I wanted an interview. That wouldn't be hard. I'd just call up her Harpo production company in Chicago and . . .

Not so fast.

In each city, I was told, Oprah only did interviews with national press or the station that carried her show. I guess I could understand limiting the access, but to the *Star*? That was nuts.

We may not be the *New York Times*, but we're not the *Hooterville Gazette* either. We're a major, Pulitzer Prize–winning newspaper with more than a million readers a week. I argued my case with the woman at Harpo. No luck.

I couldn't believe it. The queen of daytime was coming to my town, and they shot me down? Oh, I don't think so. I had to find another way.

I played my trump card. Years ago one of Oprah's guests had Tourette Syndrome. It comforted me to know I wasn't alone, that I wasn't just a freak. I called the Harpo lady back.

"If you won't let me interview Oprah, would you mind if I said thank you to Oprah for helping change my life?" I said. Then I read her a heartfelt note I scrawled out on a napkin over lunch. Suitably moved, the woman told me she'd let me read it to Oprah before she spoke. But to be honest, I had an ulterior motive. Once I was with her, I figured, I might be able to slip in a few reporter questions for my story.

Oprah appeared in a large Kansas City park. When the big day arrived I was taken to a small line outside a large tent, which served as a greenroom. I waited with a crew from *Entertainment Tonight* and a reporter from a local TV station.

I felt like a kid waiting to see Santa. When it was finally my turn I was ushered into the tent where I saw Oprah in a banana-yellow top holding court. She had an air about her that commanded attention. It was like nothing I had ever seen—and I've covered presidents, super-stars, and Nobel laureates. I introduced myself, shook her hand, and thanked her for taking time to see me. Seeing Oprah in person, two feet away, reminded me of how I felt when I visited all the famous sights of Washington, DC. I'd seen them on TV for years and knew they were real. But nothing could have prepared me for how I felt when I actually saw them in person.

I promised myself I'd remember everything—her smoky brown eyes, perfectly coiffed brown hair, yellow sweater tied loosely around her shoulders over a yellow striped shirt.

But at the moment, all I could think was, *Don't you move. Don't you shake.* Not now.

And then, standing directly in front of her, she turned to look at me.

"Hi, I'm Oprah Winfrey," she said with a welcoming smile on her face. Unlike other big celebrities, she didn't seem rushed or the least bit annoyed that I was taking up her valuable time. And she looked me directly in the eye.

I smiled, stuck out my hand, and tried to keep my head still. "My name's Jim Fussell," I said. "And I know you must have heard this plenty of times, but I'll only get to say it once, and it's important to me that you hear it. A long time ago you helped change my life in ways you can't possibly understand. And I just wanted to say thank you."

"*Ohhh,*" she said sweetly, as if to say, "That's really nice."

While asking her the reporter questions didn't pan out, the heart-felt-thank-you part went better than I could have expected. I told her about my Tourette's and how her shows had helped me. Then, as if on cue, my head shook hard to the left, then harder still back to the

right. I told myself I wouldn't cry, but several times I had to blink
back the tears.

I had come so far. I was forty-six years old, married, successful,
happy. I had two wonderful children. And though it continued to attack
me every day, my Tourette's had not won. And here, in front of me, was
one of the reasons why. Whether talking about people with Tourette's
or about people living with other forms of adversity, I realized that her
show—and Oprah herself—had been an inspiration to me.

She was clearly moved by my words—so much so that when I finished thanking her, she threw her arms around me and gave me a great
big hug.

Here's the thing about being hugged by Oprah Winfrey. You don't
really appreciate it when it's happening. You're too busy going, *Omigod!
Omigod! Omigod!* I hadn't asked for the hug. And as a reporter who was
supposed to remain objective and dispassionate, it left me a tad uncomfortable. On the other hand, who cared? Oprah hugged me. It was cool.
Most of all it just shocked the hell out of me.

Things like this just don't happen in my life. Oprah Winfrey is
the most powerful person in show business, a billionaire who changes
people's lives the way other people change their socks. And I was—well,
I was nobody. But there I was, face-to-face with her, telling her about
my life, about my pain, about my struggles. And she was listening, nodding, looking me in the eyes like she not only understood but actually
cared. And then she smiled that warm, welcoming Oprah smile, her
eyes softened, and she moved toward me with open arms.

What could I do?

In twenty years as a reporter I had covered my share of famous people—Ronald Reagan, Bill Clinton, Archbishop Desmond Tutu, movie
stars, billionaires. I hadn't hugged one of them. But I have to say the hug
from Oprah was nice—warm, with a squeeze in the middle. But it was
weird too. As we pulled back, I heard the crowd chanting for her, their
voices thundering through the park like a herd of bison.

"O-PRAH! O-PRAH! O-PRAH! O-PRAH!"

I had just hugged an international billionaire, and one of the most
popular and powerful people on the planet. A chill ran down my spine. I
would have been happy to walk away without another word. And other
celebrities would have let me. Oprah wanted to do more.

"Did you see my medical miracles show?" she asked.

"I'm sorry," I said. "I missed that one."

Oprah looked aghast. "You didn't see Jeff Matovic?" she said, as if everybody else had.

Jeff who? I thought. "I'm sorry," I said. "I must have missed that one."

"Oh!" she said, as if I had missed the biggest opportunity of my life. "We've got to get you the tape of Jeff Matovic." Oprah turned to address a group of assistants flitting around the tent.

"We've got to get Jim the tape of Jeff Matovic. GET JIM THE TAPE OF JEFF MATOVIC!" As they began scurrying around, nearly bumping into each other, Oprah turned back to me and winked. "We'll send you the tape."

"What's on it?" I asked.

She flashed a knowing smile that seemed to say, "You'll see."

13

Hope in the Mail

WEEKS LATER, AS I was shooting baskets in the driveway of my home in the Kansas City suburb of Lenexa, Kansas, my eleven-year-old daughter, Allison, walked up with an armload of mail.

"What's Harpo?" she asked, reading the markings on a thickly padded envelope.

"Hmmm?" I said, running after a high-arcing shot that bounced hard off the back of the rim and out toward Allie on a hot August day.

"It's on this package for you," she said. "It says Harpo Studios." She handed me the package. "What is it?" she asked.

I dropped the ball.

"It's from . . . *Oprah Winfrey*," I said, as my mind raced back to my recent encounter with the talk show maven.

"Daddy, why was there a package from Oprah Winfrey in our mailbox?"

"This is the tape!" I said, feeling the hard rectangular shape inside the package. "I forgot! She said she was going to send it to me."

"Send you what?"

"Oh, it's just something she wanted me to see, sweetie," I said. "Medical miracle or something."

Allie shrugged her shoulders.

"Bo-ring," she said, running back toward the house.

I tore open the brown package and read the label on the side of the tape. The Oprah Winfrey Show: Radical Medical Makeovers. Original airdate 4/21/04.

I walked back toward the court and set the tape on a flat landscape rock as I finished my shooting workout with a few layups and twenty free throws.

"What's that?" my wife asked, nodding to the envelope on the rock as she walked past with our overloaded recycling bin. "It's actually from Oprah Winfrey," I said, taking the green bin from her and walking it to the curb.

"Thanks," she said as she as she walked alongside me. "Did you say Oprah?"

"Yeah," I said. "It's my tape."

"Your *tape*?" she said. "Since when does the *Oprah* show send *you* tapes?"

"It's not from the *Oprah show*," I said, correcting her. "It's from Oprah Winfrey herself!"

"Oh-kay," she said, rolling her eyes. "Since when does Oprah Winfrey send you tapes?"

"She said she'd send it, and *she did*!"

Susan looked at me in the quizzical way I imagine her preschoolers sometimes look at her.

"And Oprah is sending you a tape from one of her shows because . . . ?"

"Actually I had forgotten about it."

"*Because?*"

"You know, this is very impressive. Most people who promise to send you things never do."

"*BE-CAUSE?*"

"I don't know," I said, setting the bin down on the edge of the grass and turning to walk back. "Because she . . . thought it was important for some reason."

"What's on it?"

"I don't know."

"Let's put it in!" she said, picking up the package.

I snatched it back from her just as fast. "I'll . . . watch it later," I said, setting it back on the rock.

"Why not just put it in now?" she said. "I'm curious to see what she sent you. We can *all* see it."

"Later," I said, bouncing the ball and swishing a twenty-foot jumper. "Why do you care so much?"

She flashed me her best "What are you, stupid?" face. "It's not every day my husband gets something from Oprah Winfrey!" she said.

"I guess I'm just full of surprises," I said, smiling and puffing out my chest as I did a little happy dance in front of her.

"You're full of *something*," she said, shaking her head and going back inside.

After I finished shooting I laid the brown package on the top of our oak entertainment center and got a glass of ice water.

Susan, a longtime Oprah fan, made a beeline for the tape. "OK, it's later," she said, slipping it into the VCR.

"No!" I said, taking it out.

"You're not going to watch it?"

"I want to watch it by myself," I said. "Later. *A lot* later."

"Why?"

"It's just . . . personal. You know?"

I stuffed the tape under my shirt and took it down to the basement.

"Jim?"

In the furnace room I hid it deep in a cardboard box of painting drop cloths under my workbench.

"Jim?"

"Yeah?" I said, jogging back up.

"I want to see it sometime."

"You will," I said.

Later that night, an hour after everyone had gone to bed, I sat on the beige carpet in the middle of our darkened family room with a bowl of salted peanuts and a glass of skim milk and slipped the tape into the VCR.

There are moments that are so powerful you realize in an instant they're going to change your life. For me, watching the tape of Jeff Matovic was one of those moments. The tape showed Jeff before his surgery, tortured and imprisoned by a horrible case of Tourette's. I saw him writhe and shake and have trouble completing a simple sentence. I saw him try to walk down a hallway, only to be interrupted by electric spasms that caused him to stop to twitch and shake. Even though my Tourette's was nowhere near as strong, I understood all too well what he was going through. In the next clip I saw Jeff after his surgery. Then, unbelievably, I saw him walk across the stage with his wife, Debra, to thunderous applause.

I couldn't move. I literally sat there with my mouth open.

"That's impossible!" I said. "Nobody just beats Tourette Syndrome like that!" And yet, there he was—the man who had done it.

In that moment I knew that everything I had ever believed about the invincibility of Tourette Syndrome was wrong. It *wasn't* permanent! It *wasn't* all-powerful! It didn't have to define or destroy my future!

I rewound the tape. Then I rewound it again. I copied down Jeff's name and began to cry. I paused the tape on a close-up of Jeff's face and scooted in closer to reach out and touch it with a trembling hand. I watched him twitch and jerk, flex, and flail, his body a Gordian knot of spasms. It was awful, but I couldn't look away. My heart went out to him—and to his family. The things they must have been through! The embarrassment. The frustration. The exhaustion and the pain.

No one could know the depths of their despair—not even me. But I knew one thing: I've interviewed thousands of people, and the more I learned about Jeff Matovic, I knew he was different from all of them. He easily had led the most courageous, awful, and wonderful life I had ever seen.

It wasn't long before I knew what I had to do. I had to meet Jeff Matovic. I had to meet—as Oprah called him—the Miracle Man! And at that moment I knew I would. In many ways I had been searching for Jeff my whole life. He represented every crazy, miraculous possibility I ever dreamed might come true. More important, he represented the one thing I thought I'd never have again with my Tourette's. He represented hope.

The next day I called Eileen Korey, head of public relations at the hospital where Jeff had his surgery. Lots of people wanted a piece of Jeff after that show. It was Eileen's job to keep most of them away—or at least that's how it seemed to me. But after hearing that I had Tourette's myself, she agreed to give me his number. I wrote it down on a yellow legal pad. I ripped out the page and looked at the numbers. A chill ran up my back. I was about to talk to a man who had triumphed over his Tourette's, a man I had convinced myself couldn't exist. And if could just work up the nerve, I was going to fly to Cleveland to meet him and ask him if I could write a book about his life.

Just the thought of it was exciting, energizing. Although I didn't know it then, I was holding more than a telephone number in my hands.

I was holding my future.

I said a prayer, picked up the receiver, and—with trembling hands—dialed the number.

"Hello?" Jeff said in a deep voice on the other end of the line.

"Jeff?" I said, fidgeting and cradling the phone with two hands as if it might break if I dropped it. "This is Jim Fussell from Kansas City. Do you . . . have a few minutes?"

"Of course," Jeff said.

The voice on the other end of the line—my voice—was breathless, apologetic.

I spoke quickly in short, choppy sentences. I was a forty-six-year-old professional, but in some ways I must have sounded like a schoolgirl.

"I—I—I hope I didn't disturb you," I stammered.

"No, it's fine," Jeff said. "I was just watching a track meet on TV and eating some nachos. I've got the afternoon free."

I took a deep breath and blew it out. I told Jeff I was a writer with Tourette Syndrome. I told him about Oprah and the tape and how I couldn't believe what I had seen. I told him how amazing his story was, and how it had given me hope. And, with trembles of emotion in my voice, I told him that he was my hero.

"I've interviewed presidents, movie stars, billionaires, and Nobel Prize winners. But it would be one of the biggest honors of my life if I could get on a plane and fly to Cleveland to meet you. Would that be OK?"

"Of course," he told me.

Talking to Jeff gave me goose bumps the size of marbles. He was just like me. No. He was *better* than me. He had not just survived Tourette's, he had beaten it! To me, he might as well have been a rock star. The only disappointing part of the conversation was the date of our meeting. Because of all the things that were going on in his life, he couldn't meet with me until late fall.

I took what I could get.

In early November 2004, I boarded a plane from Kansas City to Cleveland to meet Jeff for the first time. Because of the extra stress flying puts on my head, it's not my favorite thing to do—especially if the plane is delayed and I can't get off and move around.

Guess what? The plane was delayed and I couldn't get off and move around.

I spent as much time as I could in the tiny bathroom. But soon they wanted everyone back in their seats, buckled up and ready to go. I felt like a prisoner. It wasn't long before my head started to rebel. I felt like a person in a coffin who had just woken up to discover that someone had made a terrible mistake. I wanted to get out of there! I started breathing hard. I closed my eyes hard and said a prayer. The constant madness inside my brain pushing at me, pressuring me to shake and twist and flex, was indescribable. I tried to fight it by counting to a thousand and doing deep breathing exercises.

It helped—at least for a while.

Soon I couldn't fight anymore. For me, holding back a shake is like holding back an eye blink. I don't care how much willpower you have, eventually it's just going to happen.

An hour into the delay my head started shaking—a lot. And I don't know if someone complained, but shortly thereafter a middle-aged flight attendant with bottle-blonde hair, a leathery tan, and a chest that looked as if it had been inflated with a gas station air hose walked up to me.

"Sir?" she said in a syrupy sweet tone.

"Yes?" I said.

"Is there anything I can do for you to make you more...comfortable?"

"No, but thanks for asking," I said, wrenching my neck hard, then grabbing it with my hand.

"Because if there's any way we could help you feel more relaxed, we would want to do that."

"I'm afraid I'm about as relaxed as I get," I said.

She looked at me again as I fought back a wave of tension, then snapped my head to the left.

"Oh, you mean my head shaking?" I said. "I've got something called Tourette Syndrome."

"Whatever you have, we just need you to stop it before we get under way," she said.

Whatever I have? Oh this was going to be interesting.

"Uhh . . . I'll try my best," I said. "But I'm afraid it doesn't work that way."

"What can we do to help you?"

"You could *take off*," I said.

"We have a pillow," she said sweetly, reaching for an unimpressive white lump.

"I really don't need a pil—"

She handed it to me.

"Yeah. OK. Thanks."

"Is there anything else we can do to help you keep perfectly still?" she asked.

I looked at the cheap pillow, then threw it in the seat next to me.

"That depends," I said. "Do you have magical powers?"

"Do I have what, sir?"

"You know, can you perform miracles? Turn water to wine? That sort of stuff."

"Excuse me?"

"You wouldn't happen to offer in-flight massages in coach, would you?"

"I'm afraid not, sir."

"Then I think we're pretty much stuck with where I'm at comfort-wise. But thanks for asking."

The flight took a couple of hours. It seemed more like a week. I didn't care.

Jeff was worth it.

14

I Have a Bazillion Questions

THERE WAS NOTHING particularly memorable about my Cleveland motel. Across the street from a busy strip mall, it could have been in any one of a hundred cities. But to me it was the most beautiful place I had ever seen. This was where I was going to meet Jeff. And I couldn't help but feel good as I walked through the door.

"*Lu*-cyyyy," I bellowed, setting down my large blue suitcase and spreading my arms wide. "I'm *ho*-ome!"

I smiled at my own joke. I was such a *dork*.

I closed the door and a surge of nervous energy shot from my stomach through my upper chest. I blinked three times, tensed the muscles in my neck, then shook my head left and right four times in a row. I was *so excited* that I was finally going to meet Jeff. Maybe too excited.

I couldn't wait to tell him I was in town. Sitting down in front of a mirror, I watched myself pick up the phone, then put it down. I stared at Jeff's number, handwritten in one of my white reporter's notebooks. I drew circles around the number, then doodled smaller circles around that. I grabbed the phone again, then put it down. Grabbed it. Put it down. I tapped my pen, popped my knuckles, then began picking at the edge of the wooden desk where the veneer had begun to peel away.

I took a breath and grabbed the phone again.

"You can do this," I said.

I set the phone back in its cradle. The adrenaline took one more lap around my chest, causing me to walk restively around the room. I realized what was about to happen. And for the first time it frightened me.

Who did I think I was? Was I really going to tell Jeff Matovic I wanted to write his book? He had just been on Oprah *and* Good Morning America. *He could get anyone to tell his story! Besides, I didn't know the first thing about writing a book.*

"Shut up!" I said out loud, trying to stop the nervous thoughts. I was a writer. A good writer. And I had one thing that all those other writers didn't.

"You might actually come in handy for once," I said, talking to my Tourette's. Digging into my black laptop briefcase I pulled out a story I had written in 1990 for *Star Magazine*, the Sunday magazine of the *Kansas City Star*, about my own Tourette's. I read a passage.

> There is no cure for Tourette Syndrome, but some drugs can lessen the severity of its symptoms. Researchers believe that Tourette's is genetic, and there is evidence it runs in families, although not in mine. In the Middle Ages such tics were seen as a sign of demonic possession. When exorcism failed to drive the spirits from the body, people were burned as witches.
>
> Today people just make fun of you.
>
> "Hey you!" a scruffy high school student yelled at me once. "Are you a spazmeister or what?"
>
> "No," I said. "I'm a reporter for the *Kansas City Star*."
>
> He flipped me his middle finger, jerked his head backward, and wiggled his body in mock contortions.
>
> "I have Tourette Syndrome," I said. "It's a medical condition."
>
> He ran off, getting high fives from his buddies. I got into my car and considered running him over.
>
> I hate people sometimes.
>
> And I hate having Tourette Syndrome.

I was ready. I picked up the phone and dialed Jeff's number.

When he answered I told him I had arrived, and excitedly asked when I could swing by his place. He seemed hesitant, cautious. After a while I got the feeling he didn't want me at his house at all.

Uh-oh. Had I scared him? Was he having second thoughts about talking to me?

Finally he proposed an alternative. He'd come to my motel—on Wednesday.

It was Monday.

Two days? I thought. *But I've come all this way. I want to see you now!*

"Uh, sure," I said. "Wednesday would be fine."

And it would, I told myself. I had the room for three days, and I needed to talk to his doctors anyway. With nothing else to do that day I crawled into bed to rest my head. Stressed from the flight, I fell into a deep sleep for what seemed like the first time in a month.

I awoke past 9:00 PM to a gurgling stomach. In all the excitement I had forgotten to eat. I drove across a busy street into a strip mall, where I ordered a large beef sandwich from a neighborhood pub and took it back to my room.

Sitting on the bed with the white Styrofoam takeout container in my lap, I turned on the TV to a nice surprise: my favorite team, the Philadelphia Eagles, were playing their hated rivals the Dallas Cowboys on *Monday Night Football*. And they were winning. Big.

I took that as a good sign as I cheered and ran around the room. As I finished off the sandwich, the Eagles finished off the Cowboys 49–21.

"Maybe this is going to work out after all," I said to myself.

━ ━

ACROSS TOWN, JEFF wasn't so sure. He didn't know me. And while he *wanted* to believe I was the right person to write his book, that was far from guaranteed.

More than anything, he was tired. Tired of the excitement and the shows and the white-hot media blitz. He was tired of the opportunists and the glad-handers and the people who were using him for their own purposes. He longed for someone who could truly understand him.

Late Wednesday afternoon he tried to relax before making the nervous twenty-minute drive to my motel. And there was nothing that relaxed him more than listening to his favorite comedian, Jeff Foxworthy.

He popped in a DVD and flopped on the couch. He knew each joke
by heart. Like a good friend, they never got old. There was something
about Foxworthy's singsong Southern drawl that got Jeff every time.

Jeff looked at the screen. A smiling Foxworthy was in the middle
of his famous "You Might Be a Redneck" routine, and the audience was
roaring.

"If you've been married three times and still have the same in-
laws," Foxworthy said. "You might be a redneck."

Stretched out on his back, Jeff couldn't help but smile.

Half an hour later he was dressed and ready to walk out the door.

"How do I look?" he asked his wife.

"Very handsome," she said.

"Thanks," he said, smiling and giving her a kiss. "You're not so bad
yourself." He started out the door, then stopped. The smile was gone.

"What is it, babe?" Debra asked.

Jeff looked back at his wife. "I just hope he's someone I can hit it
off with and really talk to," he said. "I know this could be a great book.
But I need someone who really understands me, and also understands
the condition."

Debra gave him an "I know" with her eyes.

"Say a prayer for me," Jeff said. "It's not often you meet someone
with Tourette's, let alone a guy not much older than I am who just happens to be a feature writer for a large newspaper."

"I'm sure you two will hit it off just fine," Debra said.

As he drove through familiar streets he played the radio loudly,
tapping wildly on the steering wheel to the driving rock beat. When he
arrived, he turned off the engine but didn't get out of the car. He took a
big breath, closed his eyes, and offered a prayer.

"God," he said, "let this be the person I need."

BACK AT THE motel I grew nervous as the minutes to our meeting
ticked down.

Twenty minutes before Jeff arrived, I carefully laid out on the desk
all the stories I had brought to share with him. I set them out as if in a
display.

No. Trying too hard, I thought, quickly putting them back in a pile. I combed my hair, practiced various greetings in front of the mirror, and changed clothes three times.

He *had* to like me, he just had to. He had to know how much he had inspired me and given me hope. He had to understand why I was the perfect one to write a book about his life, and why no one could care more. What words could I use to convince him? I knelt in front of the king-sized bed and bowed my head. Five minutes later the knock at the door might as well have been the beating of my heart.

I opened it to reveal a tall man with black hair wearing a large and friendly smile. Looking exactly as he had on TV, he extended his hand.

"Jeff Matovic," he said with a huge grin.

"I recognize you from the tape," I said. "Jim Fussell. Come on in and sit down."

I sat at the desk. Jeff, dressed in a green polo, khaki shorts, and brown sandals, sat across from me on the edge of the bed.

I liked him immediately. He was funny, smart, and kind. And it didn't take long to figure out that we had faced the same demons. We finished each other's sentences and fit like puzzle pieces. My eyes lit up every time I heard him say something about his life that paralleled something in mine. We began to laugh, trade stories, and excitedly interrupt each other.

"Have you ever been in the situation where . . ."

"Oh! Oh! And what about when your tics . . ."

"And how about when you do this . . ." I said making my neck motion.

"Yeah!" Jeff said. "Or this," he said, making a movement of his own.

"I know *exactly* what you mean!" I'd say. And I did.

It was as if Jeff and I had known each other forever. The conversation was organic and cathartic. He told me about the time he scared a little old lady when he had a particularly violent tic just as the doors opened on an elevator. He told me about the time he dented his dining room wall with his moving head. I hung on every word.

He felt like the brother I never had. But he was so much more. Not only was he someone who had experienced all the tics, travails, and torture of Tourette's, he was someone who had survived them and broken through to the other side.

"Sure," I said.

"Would you mind if I . . . took off my shirt?" he said, throwing up his hands as if to say, "Nothing weird or anything."

"No problem," I said.

Jeff removed his shirt and put his fingers on top of two subtle but noticeable rectangular bulges under the skin on both pecs.

"These are my batteries," he said. "They power my stimulators. Here, you can feel them."

I hesitated. It was a bit weird, but then I thought, *That's the miracle. That's what helped him be normal and to defeat his tics.*

I put my hand on the chest bulge and felt the hard battery below. "Does it hurt?"

"No," he said. "I can't even feel it. These are connected to a very thin wire that runs up to the stimulators in my brain."

He turned his head and craned his neck.

"It's small, but you can see if you look closely."

I could see the outline of the wire—barely—running up the side of his long neck.

"Wow!" I said. "That is unreal!"

"Isn't it?"

"That is so cool. And that . . ."

"Powers the stimulators in my brain that control my tics."

My mouth just hung open. Seeing it in person, that close up, made shivers run down my spine. Maybe I could have that same surgery one day! Maybe I could get better.

Maybe.

It was almost like adult show-and-tell. I read him my articles; he showed me his batteries and his wires. It was one of the most remarkable moments of my life. In the two hours we had been together he already had become an important friend and partner, the brother I never had, and the hero I always needed.

Near the end of the meeting I thanked Jeff for coming and told him how incredible it was to meet him. Then I pressed my case, listing reasons why I would be the perfect person to write his book. Jeff told me my passion, enthusiasm, humor, storytelling, and personal familiarity with Tourette's was everything he could have wanted in an author. Still, when I asked him if we could write the book together, he was noncommittal.

I stared at him in disbelief. He wasn't moving. He wasn't suffering. He was . . . *well*!

"You know, what I told you on the phone was the truth," I said, looking him in the eye. "As corny as it sounds, you're my hero." I fought back a tear. "I never thought something like this was possible. For more than forty years this thing has tortured me—not as badly as it tortured you, but it's bad enough."

Jeff saw my tics. He also saw my passion and sensed my integrity. Tourette's was not just some subject I found interesting. It was the biggest part of me, affecting me in some way in every moment of my life.

Jeff listened to the way I talked about the condition, about my experiences. He saw the look of recognition in my eyes when he talked about his experiences. And he felt my heart when I told him, again, how inspirational his story was, that he was my hero, and that I would be honored to write a book with him.

Jeff thought about how I hadn't just called him and asked him to write the book, but actually spent my own money to come to see him in Cleveland. That put a checkmark in my column. He told me later that my genuineness, my integrity, and my work ethic reminded him of his father.

Finally the time for talking was done. I wanted Jeff to know what kind of a writer I was.

"I brought some articles that I've written so you can get a sense of how I write," I said. "Would you mind if I read them?"

"No," Jeff said. "I'd love to hear them."

I grabbed the article on the top of the pile—a story I had written in the *Kansas City Star* in the fall of 1993 about the time my daughter, Allison, was born at home on the bed. I read it to Jeff.

"That's an amazing story, and beautifully written," Jeff said.

"Thank you," I said.

"I felt like I was there. And I just can't believe you did that!"

"Yeah," I said. "Neither can I."

"Could I read you another one?"

"Absolutely," Jeff said. "This is great."

Jeff loved to hear me read. He told me so. Sharing my personal stories in my own voice meant a lot to him. Later, Jeff shared something even more personal with me.

"You want to see something cool?" he said.

"It's been great talking," he said. "But as excited as we are, we need to come down from the high we're on. We'll talk about this in a couple of days."

Worried, I asked if there was anyone else who had begun work on the story. He paused, and then looked down.

My heart sank. *No!*

He already had started working with another author.

I hung my head. I had come all that way, poured my heart out, and bonded with a man with an incredible story only to find out that somebody else was writing the book I was born to write. Sensing my disappointment, Jeff tried to broker a compromise.

"I don't see any reason there couldn't be two books," he said. "The other one is coming from a little different angle, dealing more with the psychological realm. Would you be OK with that?"

"Uh . . . I guess," I said, halfheartedly, not wanting to lose my chance at his story. But deep down I knew I'd have to tell Jeff that there could only be one book about his amazing story.

Jeff moved toward the door. Time to go. We shook hands.

At that moment I also knew something else—that *I was going to be the one to write it*! I had always played fair. I never wanted to hurt people or get something I didn't deserve. But in this case I had to be competitive. And I wanted to win! I felt badly about being a claim jumper, about causing someone else to lose their dream in order for me to get mine. But this was far too important to me to feel too badly for too long.

I didn't mind competing. And I thought I could win. Sure, the other author had a head start. But I had an ace in the hole. I had *Tourette's.*

Finally I got some good news. The other author had barely started a couple of weeks ago, and Jeff didn't exactly seem to have an unbreakable relationship with him. In fact, Jeff was still trying to understand and bond with the author, telling him one thing but wondering privately if it was worth continuing. He was a little dry, Jeff later told me. And he didn't feel that same spark of life that he did with me.

"I can't wait to get started on the book," I said. "I have a bazillion questions!"

"I have a bazillion stories," he said.

His wide smile seemed to say that, one way or another, this book was going to happen.

"Yes!" I vowed. "It will happen."

After Jeff left, I waited several minutes to make sure he was out of earshot, and then checked the parking lot to make sure. Then, I couldn't control my excitement any longer. Everything I had been keeping inside of me for more than forty years—all the pain, all my struggles, all my hopes and dreams, came rushing out of me all at once. I began running in circles in the hotel room, exploding with laughter, tears, shouts of joy, and primal screams. I danced on the table, jumped on the dresser, and nearly broke my arm trying to do a backward somersault off the bed from my knees.

It was easily one of the greatest moments of my life. I felt as if I had been reborn, or at least plugged into an electrical outlet. The power surge racing through my body was unlike anything I have ever felt. I had just met the walking embodiment of my wildest dream—living proof that every fear I ever had about never being able to get better was just *meaningless bullshit*! I didn't care if they ever did deep brain stimulation on people with less serious cases like mine. Just the fact that they had done it on one person, and it had worked, was more than enough for me. I knew now that my Tourette's was mortal. It could be stopped.

It could be *killed*!

It wouldn't happen overnight. It might never happen. But just knowing that it was possible gave me enough energy to run a marathon—or at least around the hotel several times, which I did with a huge grin on my face. Finally winded, I stopped in the parking lot to catch my breath. When I did, I saw a license plate on the back of a cherry-red mustang. It read CELEBR8.

I looked up in the sky, and pointed. "Try and stop me," I said.

15

"What Are You, Stupid, Matovic?"

WHEN I GOT home I felt like Superman. Energy radiated from every pore. Usually I was tired and achy. But after talking to Jeff, I felt as if I could lift a Land Rover over my head. Jeff was a hundred times more inspiring in person than he was on TV. There was so much more to his story than even I had realized. And I couldn't wait to tell it to the world.

It all seemed so right. Jeff and me. The book. A story about a person with Tourette's written by a person with Tourette's. How perfect was that?

Still, there was a problem. The other book.

I didn't want another book. It was the worm in an otherwise perfect apple. After stewing over it for a couple of days, I decided to call Jeff and tell him the hard truth. There could only be one successful book about his story, and he'd have to decide who would write it. It was a risky gambit. All or nothing.

"If you feel your story would be better served with me," I told Jeff. "I would be honored beyond words. But if you feel like you should stay with the other author, I understand. He's already started. That's only fair."

I meant it. But when I hung up I had a sick feeling that I was a phone call away from losing the biggest opportunity of my life— writing a book about a person who had given my daily struggle a higher purpose. I knew if I let this chance slip away, another like it would not come along. If I ever was going to write a book, this was it. After hanging up I folded my hands and closed my eyes. I had always known the difference between right and wrong, but now I was confused. Both decisions felt "right" to me in different ways.

Help us, I prayed. *Guide us to do the right thing—whatever that is.*

Two days later Jeff called back. It felt like a month. I picked up the receiver. Worried that he could hear my heart pounding through the phone, I covered the mouthpiece with my hand.

Please, God, I thought.

After a brief greeting there was a pause on the other end. Dead silence for several seconds. And then—"I talked it over with Deb," Jeff said in a measured voice. "And . . . we would be honored if you would be the one to write the book."

I exhaled all the air that I had been holding in my chest in one big blow. "Are you sure?" I said, suddenly breathing hard. "I mean, that's wonderful . . . thank you. Umm. Thank you."

I wanted to scream.

"I'm just so glad to hear that," I said. "But . . . I mean—"

"What?" Jeff said.

"What about the other author?" I said. "I kind of feel bad now."

"Don't," he said. "I wasn't sure that it was working out anyway. I feel much more of a connection with you. And I love your writing. And, hey—I know you understand me."

I closed my eyes. My dream was coming true. I was going to be an author! I felt energized, focused, *alive!*

Over the next half hour Jeff and I talked excitedly about our hopes and dreams for the book and made plans for nightly interviews. When I hung up I jumped in the air and pumped my fist, landing with a loud boom on the dining room floor. "*Yes!*" I shouted.

My father always dreamed of writing a book, but never did—unless you count a short autobiography that he bound himself. He would have been so proud of me. At the same time I had a different emotion that I hadn't counted on: fear.

This certainly was a great opportunity. It also was a *huge* responsibility. And now that Jeff had chosen me, I wondered, could I really write a book? I knew I'd need hundreds more hours of interviews if it was going to be any good. I knew we'd need a publishing company. Beyond that I knew nothing. Less than nothing. I didn't even know what I didn't know.

"I can learn," I said under my breath.

I defaulted to what I knew as a reporter—a steady diet of interviewing and transcribing. We began talking after work and on the weekends, slowly peeling back the layers of his fascinating life. I wanted to go quickly. Unfortunately I had Ferrari ambitions with a Yugo motor. After patchy sleep and ticking my way through a full day at work, I could only go so fast.

I had done in-depth interviewing before, but nothing like this. Jeff's story was deep, like the rabbit hole in *Alice in Wonderland*. And the more I learned about the story, the deeper the hole went.

ONE OF THE most interesting parts of our first interview concerned Jeff's years in grade school, when strange movements began to take hold of his body. Plenty of kids teased him, but none did it better than a charming antagonist named Ron.

Jeff met Ron in first grade at St. Bonaventure, a parochial school in Glenshaw, Pennsylvania. Rich, entitled, smart, cool, arrogant, and mean, there was a suave charisma to Ron that attracted followers like a magnet. He was a good seven inches shorter than Jeff, but what he lacked in height he more than made up for in confidence and ego. Ron was a bully and a button pusher, and if he didn't like you, you became his target.

Not even his teachers were immune. If a teacher stumbled over a word, Ron would be the first to laugh. Even when a teacher would threaten to send him to the office, he wouldn't break character.

"Yeah," he'd fire back with a sneer on his face, "like I haven't done *that* before!"

Jeff met Ron's parents once. They were permissive, gave him whatever he wanted, tried to be his best friend. They spoiled him.

Jeff couldn't have been more different. Polite, kind, and respectful, Jeff would try to make peace with Ron. When insulted or teased, Jeff would try to lighten the mood with a joke, or just leave without making the situation worse.

Ron interpreted Jeff's good manners as weakness. He didn't like Jeff. He had found his target.

IT WAS LUNCHTIME at St. Bonaventure grade school. Jeff slid a cafeteria tray along three silver bars that served as a guide rail. The tallest kid in school, he was a big eater. He loaded his tray with a sloppy joe, four cartons of milk, and double helpings of mac and cheese, mashed potatoes and gravy, and chocolate chip cookies. Before Jeff reached the cashier, Ron reached under his tray and poked it from the bottom, causing all his food to spill. Then he pointed at Jeff.

"What are you, stupid, Matovic?" he said. "You have to keep the food on the plate to eat it!" And then everyone in the lunchroom would laugh.

Jeff hated it when he spilled the food on his lunch tray. Sometimes it was because of Ron; other times because his tics. Most days he tried to scoot the tray along, touching it only briefly. As he moved along the line, collecting food, a powerful urge grew in his right arm—the urge to punch hard, straight down. Day after day it built to overwhelming levels until—oh God!—he simply had to punch downward, and he had to do it *right then*!

Jeff's long arm fired downward like a backward missile—hard, fast, straight down. As it did, a tremendous clatter echoed through the lunchroom. His rocket arm had clipped the front of his lunch tray on the way down, sending his food—including a plate covered in brown gravy, all over the front of his carefully pressed white shirt.

Everyone turned to look. Immediately after, he could hear Ron's derisive voice pierce the uncomfortable silence. "Hey, Matovic!" he called. "Did you bring an extra set of clothes today? Did you bring your *diaper*?"

Ron burst out laughing. Other times he'd just stand and applaud, or lean back in his chair with a knowing smirk. It was like a private victory for him whenever Jeff's tics would embarrass him. When Jeff would look over, Ron would just smile and wink. Jeff felt like a big joke. Just another of Ron's punch lines.

But in another way, Ron motivated Jeff. He made him resolved and focused. Jeff wanted nothing more than to put the charming asshole in his place. And as they grew older, that's just what he did. One day in 1984, when Jeff was in fifth grade, he had gone out for recess with his best friends, Kevin Keenan, Dan Kenaan, and Pat Rios. Ron and his posse were playing hoops, and Ron was showing off.

A good athlete, Ron hit a few long shots, causing his admirers to say "Wow!" When he saw Jeff, Ron said, "Let me show you something I can do that Matovic could *never* do."

Dribbling twice between his legs, Ron did a 360-degree spin and fired up a three-pointer that dropped into the net.

"*Ooohhhh!*" said his posse.

Ron stared Jeff down with his arms spread wide. "What you got?" he said in a challenging voice.

Dan put his hand on Jeff's shoulder. "It ain't even worth it," he said.

"No," Jeff said, walking toward Ron. "I need to take care of something. Gimmie the ball!" he said to Ron.

Jeff not only imitated Ron's move, he dribbled the ball between his legs five times, did two spins and—while fading to his left from a greater distance than from where Ron shot—threw the ball up in a high arc. Perfect swish.

Ron's friends wore a look of shock as they stared at Jeff.

After retrieving the ball, Jeff forcefully pushed it into Ron's chest and then walked away.

Kevin, Dan, and Pat had smiles a mile wide. "Holy crap," Kevin said. "That was incredible! Did you know you could make that?"

"Nope," Jeff said with a crooked smile. "Guess it's good to be lucky sometimes."

———

BUT JEFF SAVED the best for last. Seventh grade. Spring 1986. All sixth, seventh, and eighth graders were outside for a field day called the "Grand Olympics." There were running and throwing and jumping events. The prizes: red, white, and blue ribbons and bronze, silver, and gold foil-wrapped chocolate coins that melted quickly in the summer sun.

Jeff came in first in numerous events, even beating many eighth graders. Finally, he reached the last, and most prestigious, event of the day: the 100-meter dash. Jeff toed the chalk starting line. He looked beside him to see his challenger. Ron grinned back at him.

"I'm taking this from you, Matovic," he said.

"Go ahead and try," Jeff said.

At the sound of the gun there was enough cheering that—for Jeff—it might as well have been the Olympics. His legs drove hard off the line as he pulled out to a quick lead. Knees pumping, arms swinging, and lungs puffing like a locomotive, he flew across the finish line a good fifteen yards ahead of Ron.

As Ron panted, Jeff looked at his vanquished rival with a satisfied smile. "Ron?" he said. "You need a drink?"

Suddenly silent, Ron turned and walked away. Kevin and Dan ran up and jumped on their friend.

"I can't believe how fast you were," Kevin said. "That was amazing! I've never seen anyone run that fast in my life!"

That weekend Jeff played in a basketball game. His parents watched from the stands with Kevin and Dan. In between plays they watched him stand on the court and tic uncontrollably, kicking his legs, punching his arms and grunting loudly.

"*Huh! Huh!*"

Just then a kid a couple rows in front of them began making fun of Jeff—mocking his movements, laughing, and calling him names.

Kevin had heard enough. "Knock it off!" he screamed at the kid. "He has a problem, and the doctor's trying to find the medicine." That shut the kid up. Jeff's mother had never been prouder of Kevin that at that moment.

That night, as they often did, Jeff and Kevin slept over at Dan's house. As usual, they played games, watched TV, and talked all night. The subject of Ron, and how Jeff had smoked him in the race, dominated much of the conversation. In the morning Dan and Kevin told Jeff not to pay any attention to Ron's cruel taunts, and that he was just jealous.

"Guys," Jeff said with a large arm punch and leg kick before leaving to go home, "I don't care about people making fun of me like Ron does. I just need to learn how to survive without you guys."

Kevin looked down and shook his head. "Gonna miss you like hell, Matovic," he said, giving Jeff a fist bump.

"Big time," said Dan.

16

Comfort from Katie

JEFF RETURNED FROM the sleepover looking as if he had lost his best friend. His eyes were red, his lips pursed.

"What's wrong, dear heart?" his mother asked.

He looked down. He knew this was the last sleepover he would ever have with Kevin and Dan. Several months earlier his father had given him the bad news. He had been transferred. They were moving to Cleveland.

It was February 1986, a month after his thirteenth birthday, in the middle of his seventh-grade year.

"I know it's hard," his mother said, putting her arm around him.

Such news would upset any child. But for Jeff it was doubly difficult. Life had improved since he found the courage to talk to Kevin and Dan about his tics. They had become an invaluable part of his support system. He couldn't envision life without them. After the bad news, Jeff had gone through stages. He had reasoned, protested, shouted, and cried.

Why does Dad have to be in the steel industry? he thought. *Why can't he just find another job with computers? Why can't he just stay here? There have got to be other things here.*

He begged his dad. "Isn't there something else you can find?"

It was no use. They were moving. And there was nothing he could do about it but get mad. After school and on weekends he'd throw a baseball against their dark green shed, then throw a football as hard as he could against the brick part of the house.

Finally, he had to accept his fate. His mother and father knew how difficult this was for their boys. They tried their best to make it up to them.

"Come on," his mother said later than evening, as a glum Jeff walked past her in the living room. "Let's go out and get some ice cream!"

Jeff shook his head no. Then he shook it from side to side.

"Are you sure, honey?" she asked in her sweet, comforting voice. "Your dad and I would love to treat you to the movies today. It will be dark, there will be air conditioning. How does that sound?"

Jeff was conflicted. One part of him really wanted to see a movie. But another part—the one with Tourette's—sounded a warning.

Everyone's going to be looking at you, you freak!

"Mom," Jeff said, stooping to pick up the family dog, "I don't want to go anywhere. I'll just stay home with Katie."

Katie was an eighteen-pound black cockapoo with three white paws and a white stripe under her neck which ran down to her belly. She was the first pet Jeff had really loved. Even if he was having a horrible day, Katie could always make things better. Katie was not allowed on the furniture.

One night, before the move to Cleveland, he asked his mother for an exception. "I'm just having a really tough time with the Tourette's," he said. "Can Katie sleep with me?"

His mother looked at her youngest boy and gave a soft smile. "Absolutely," she said.

That night Katie snuggled up to Jeff. There were things he could tell Katie that he couldn't tell anyone else. He'd hold her closely, stroke her softly curled black fur, and whisper his secret frustrations in her ear. Katie trusted Jeff. When he'd finish petting her, she'd gaze up at him and paw at his hand, asking for more.

But it wasn't always like this. Weeks earlier she cowered in the corner of his room, whimpering and afraid to come near him. That was the day Jeff lost it. Katie just wanted to stay out of the way.

His explosion happened soon after he had learned that he would have to move to Cleveland. It wasn't fair! It felt like the earth was shifting under his feet, and he was being thrust into the scary unknown; like he had already run two marathons in his life and now he was back at the starting line just beginning his training. After dinner one night he told his parents he just wanted to be alone and headed for his room.

He called Katie in. She walked around the room as he stared out his bedroom window into a front yard covered in fallen snow. For a moment he felt like leaving tracks in that snow.

"I guess running away wouldn't do any good, would it Katie?" he said. He picked her up and held her in his arms. He cocked his head, feeling the softness of her ear against his. He couldn't stop thinking about the move and all the horrors it would bring. He didn't want to start again. He *couldn't* start again!

He wiped away a tear pooling in the bottom of his eye, got on his hands and knees beside his bed, and began to pray. He said some Our Fathers and some Hail Marys, but that wasn't really what he wanted to do. He was unsure what he wanted. He was just so afraid and confused and sad and mad. And then, in the middle of an Our Father he burst out sobbing.

Everything seemed to hit him all at once—leaving Pittsburgh, leaving Kevin and Dan, starting over with no support system, being the new kid, being the *weird* kid, being stressed and not knowing where to turn or who he could trust. He took his fist and starting ramming it as hard as he could on the bed saying, "No! No! No! NO!" Every hit was more forceful than the next.

Realizing he was getting loud, he stuffed his face into his pillow to muffle the sound of a scream. As his left hand pulled up the edge of the mattress, his right hand pounded away. By this time he was doing violent, full roundhouse windups with every ounce of power his six-foot body could deliver.

"It's not fair!" he screamed. "It's not fair!"

And for the first time he cursed God. "You suck!" he screamed. "I hate you! You suck! You suck! You're nothing but a letdown!" He thrashed and screamed. And when he ripped the covers off the bed, his tears soaked the bare mattress. After a few minutes he rose to his knees and ran his right hand over his aching head until he reached the back of his sweat-soaked neck. Just then he looked back at Katie to see her cowering and shaking under his desk.

Now Jeff began to cry in a different way. *Katie!*

It broke his heart to see the only pet he had ever had whimpering and afraid of him. How could he have forgotten she was in the room? He walked over to her as calmly as he could, putting his hands out as if to say "It's OK. You don't have to be afraid of me."

"Katie, it's not you," he said in a tender voice. "Come here. I love you."

He petted her until she was no longer afraid. He held her for five minutes on his bed, squeezing her softly and crying into her fur as he thought of everything that was to come.

Holding Katie calmed him down. He even laughed slightly despite himself when he saw his teardrops fall on her little black nose and onto her ears.

"Aw, I didn't mean to soak you, Katie!" he said. Gently he lifted her up under her front legs until he and his pet were face-to-face. He put his nose against hers and rubbed it.

"Katie," he said, gazing into her eyes, "at least *you're* coming with me."

17

A Teenager with Tourette's

Bay Middle School, Bay Village, Ohio. Spring 1986.

"If you're going to sleep, get out of my class!"

Everyone turned to look at Jeff.

First rule of middle school: don't call attention to yourself—especially if you're the new kid already struggling to keep people from thinking you're a freak.

Jeff didn't care. Eyelids heavy as hammers, he rested his head on his desk. When his health teacher called him on it, he lifted his head and looked at him with a blank stare.

"What?" he asked in a groggy voice.

"I said if you're going to sleep, get out of my class."

"*OK*," he mumbled, sleepily. "Where do you want me to go?"

"To the office."

"Where's that?"

"Downstairs. Take the hallway to the right. It's in the center of the hall on your left."

"Whatever," Jeff said, rising from his seat. Slouching and heavily medicated, he looked at his feet as he trudged toward the door.

For Jeff, moving to the Cleveland suburb of Bay Village in the middle of seventh grade wasn't as bad as he thought. It was worse.

Newly thirteen, he had to adjust to a new house, a new city, and a new middle school with no best friends to talk to for moral support.

Being the new kid was hard enough. But he also was the weird kid. And already over six feet, there was no place to hide.

Classmates called him Spaz Boy and Tic Man. They mocked his movements and even turned them into a dance. "Man, you are weird," they'd say, high-fiving each other as they walked away. Sometimes he just heard laughter and people asking, "What's he shaking for?"

He tried not to shake. He even took pills for it. While the powerful medication he began taking in Glenshaw just before he left reduced the frequency of his tics, too often it turned him into a zombie. He felt dull, blunted, dead inside. At its worst his brain was a slow-moving train. He didn't care if he was late for class, or even fell asleep.

Those were the bad days. He had better ones. And since he was generally a happy kid who was good at disguising his symptoms, some days there appeared to be nothing wrong with him. As a result, to many of his classmates, Jeff seemed like a walking contradiction. Was he the happy Jeff who was smart, confident, jovial, and funny—the kid who was upbeat and good in athletics? Or was he the tortured Jeff who was by turns anxious, fidgety, or zombielike—the one who often was so animated with his arms and leg movements he looked like he was playing a game of charades with himself?

That was the problem. He was both.

— —

JEFF MET HIS best friend at the end of seventh grade.

"Hey, Blair!" a boy called to a large and athletic student named Jay Blair, while motioning toward Jeff. "The new guy. You gotta arm wrestle. It'll be epic!"

A knot of middle schoolers gathered around as Blair, a blond-haired student with a big chest and thick arms, glanced toward Jeff.

Oh great, Jeff thought. He didn't want to arm wrestle anybody— especially not *that* kid. But how could he turn down such a challenge with everybody staring at him?

All right, he thought. *Let's get this over with.*

The two boys—two of the largest in school—sat down at a table in an empty classroom as a small crowd formed around them. It felt like they were in the center of a small arena. Jeff looked at Jay as they both leaned forward, set their elbows on the wooden table, and locked hands.

"Let's go," Jeff said.

"Let's go!" the kids said, roaring their approval. "Let's go!"

Jeff made a face as the match began. With a tremendous surge Jay forced Jeff's much thinner arm backward toward the table.

"Get 'em, Jay!" someone yelled. "Yeah!"

To Jay's surprise, Jeff responded with an equal surge that pulled him back to even. His arm may have been thin, but it was all muscle.

Both boys used every ounce of energy they had, trying to force the other's arm down. After several minutes of straining, their aching muscles felt as if they might explode. After nearly ten minutes both boys were drenched in sweat and staring at each other with flushed faces. Neither could win. And neither would give up.

Kids continued hooting and hollering. An exhausted Jay looked at an exhausted Jeff. "Wanna just call it a draw?" he said.

"Yeah," Jeff said, "I'm pretty tired, how 'bout you?"

"Yeah," Jay said.

They broke their grip and took big breaths as they smiled at each other and leaned back in their chairs. The crowd of kids groaned. They wanted a winner. Jay and Jeff didn't care. They had both just made a new friend.

Jay nodded at Jeff as they left the room together. He shook his arm, scrawled something on a piece of paper, and handed it to Jeff. "Here's my number," he said. "Let's get together sometime."

It wasn't long before the two became best friends. Eventually, in the summer before they went to high school, Jeff even built up enough trust to tell Jay about his Tourette's.

"That's cool, man," Jay told him. "Don't worry about it."

⌐ ¬

JEFF COULDN'T HELP but worry about it. It seemed his symptoms were getting worse every day. New tics joined with old, making them twice as terrible. Like a boxer, he moved from throwing single punches to combinations. There was eye blinking with lip smacking, head shaking with neck twisting, the sharp jab of the arm with the quick snap of the leg. And for the first time he flexed his wrists and ankles both ways, as hard as he could until it hurt, contracting his muscles and holding them so long that he wanted to cry.

At the same time puberty had begun playing its practical jokes. His cracking voice was bad enough. But when Tourette's forced him to grunt—hard enough to startle someone from across a room—it came out with a loud, embarrassing, high-pitched squeal.

Tourette's is hard at any age. But trying to be a teenager with Tourette's was like trying to fight a fire with rocket fuel. The explosive combination of becoming a teenager, being in middle school, and being a new kid while grappling with a worsening movement disorder made Jeff sometimes feel like the shoestrings of his sanity were coming untied. Most days Jeff kept his struggles to himself. But that sort of stoicism was a double-edged sword. While his ability to cope was laudable, hiding his pain only made it worse.

In the last year of middle school he didn't tell his teachers, or anybody else, that he had Tourette's. A form required to play sports asked if he had any medical conditions. He answered "none." He didn't want a piece of paper to be passed between hands of people he didn't know that in any way connected him with Tourette's.

He'd constantly wonder about that form. Was it lying face-up on a teacher's desk? What if a student saw it? What if the basketball coach pulled it out and said, "Jeff, tell me about your Tourette's and how it affects your basketball."

No. As long as he could hide it, disguise it, explain it away, or refuse to talk about it, he told himself, he would. To Jeff the letters *TS* were more than Tourette Syndrome's initials. They were scarlet letters, and he would do anything to keep from wearing them. As a result, for the first year in Bay Village, Jeff lived his life in denial. He didn't want to be a burden to his family. And he certainly didn't want to think of himself as defective or damaged.

He fought the pressure of his tics alone in his room. Screaming into his pillow became as common as combing his hair. Most mornings he cried as he looked at himself in the full-length mirror on the back of his door, trying to find the motivation to face another day. Disgusted by what he saw, he couldn't even look himself in the eyes. Many nights he went to sleep convinced he would not have the strength to get out of bed the next morning.

He always did. Thanks to his mother, he had near-perfect attendance. She would sit with him on his bed every night and cry with him. "I can't understand how hard this must be for you," she said. "For all you're going through and all you're dealing with, I just want you to remember the strength in there," she said, pointing to his head. "And in there," she said, lightly touching his chest near his heart. "And just know how much your father and I love you every day."

He nodded. He'd try, he said.

Jeff was nothing if not a good actor. He presented himself well and could fake a certain confidence that belied the pain below the surface. Tall, dark, and handsome with only a sprinkling of acne, he was a preppy dresser with a slender but athletic build. He liked to wear dark jeans and polo shirts with two T-shirts underneath for an extra-smooth appearance. He wore a gold watch and Drakkar Noir cologne and parted his short, black hair on the left, finishing with mousse and a spritz of hair spray.

Desperate not to be seen as weird, he did his best to disguise his tics, or at least delay them until he could run to the bathroom and let them out in whirlwind of uncontrollable thrashing. Letting them out felt great. Everything else felt like torture.

In high school or at the mall, no one tied his shoelaces more than Jeff. There was a reason. Sometimes, when he knew a powerful tic was coming, he would kneel and pretend to tie his shoelaces, then go into a protective turtle shell. While on one knee he would wrap his arms around his legs, lower his head, and squeeze his body together with all his strength. When the tic passed, he'd get up and go on his way.

But tics weren't his only demons. He also struggled with obsessive-compulsive disorder. It was Tourette's evil little friend. And, like his Tourette's, it only grew stronger through high school. OCD made Jeff concerned with such things as right-angle symmetry and midpoints. Everything had to be just so, or he would feel extremely uncomfortable. He had to have his schoolbooks on the upper-left-hand corner of the desk. They had to be stacked perfectly, with the biggest book on the bottom and the smallest on top. Sometimes a classmate would jostle his books or knock them to the floor to be funny. That drove Jeff crazy. He would immediately scramble to pick them up and carefully arrange them perfectly again on the upper-left corner of his desk.

Jeff's OCD did come with certain advantages. To keep from being driven crazy he had to be dressed perfectly and keep a meticulously clean and organized room. But mostly his obsessiveness caused problems— especially with schoolwork.

When he read a sentence he would have to read it over again— sometimes three or four times. Combined with his motor and vocal tics, that made homework a nightmare. Often it would take him three hours to read five pages. And sometimes a violent arm tic would cause him to rip one of those pages out of a book.

Despite the difficulty, he still got *As* in his classes. Jeff resented some of his lazier classmates who didn't know how good they had it. When a few complained about a hefty reading and writing assignment due by the end of the week, he just laughed.

You know what, you assholes? he thought. *At least you can read the book. It takes me about an hour a page. And I'm going to get it in on time, and get an* A *on it. You try doing that!*

For Jeff, fitting in at school took awhile.

But he wasn't alone. Family, friends, and classmates helped him cope. They'd read into a Dictaphone so he could hear his homework. In biology class a girl named Shannon turned the pages for him.

His guidance counselor, Miss Revnyak, was a godsend, talking him through tough times, reducing his stress, and helping him believe in his potential.

Then there was his new doctor. A world-class neurologist at the Cleveland Clinic named Gerald Erenberg took Jeff off the old medication that made him sleepy and put him on Klonopin and Orap, which helped control his tics without the sleepiness.

Erenberg was the opposite of Jeff's previous doctor. At their first meeting he smiled, put two hands on Jeff's shoulders, and looked him straight in the eye.

"We're going to do the best we can," he said. "And we're going to get you through this." He told Jeff that having Tourette's was neither his fault nor anything he could control. What's more, he helped him see that telling teachers and others that he had Tourette's would not worsen his life but drastically improve it.

In time Jeff learned that this was true. He learned to talk about his condition and even advocate for himself with teachers. One of the things he spoke to them about was his scribbled handwriting on tests.

"Obviously you are aware of my condition," he said. "If you can't read something, please ask me and I will read it to you."

His teachers agreed. One tracked him down once at lunch and said, <figure>101</figure>
"Do you have ten minutes? I'd like to review this with you." After Jeff
deciphered his scrawl, his teacher smiled.

"Cool," she said. "Thanks."

With much of his stress relieved, his natural intelligence took over.
Jeff got straight *A*s on his report card. At the end of his sophomore year
of high school he was eight for eight for the honor roll. Despite his difficulties, he was doing it. He was succeeding.

He began to think about college, even getting scholarships. And all
he wanted to do was to go back to Glenshaw, stand in front of his old
neurologist, and rub his good grades in the doctor's nose.

With the new medication helping to reduce his tics and teachers
now understanding his condition, Jeff became more confident. He made
friends, got a job at a nature center, and went on dates.

But the action that brought him the most acceptance happened in
ninth grade. Jeff had just finished his lunch in the cafeteria and was
walking toward a drinking fountain in the hall when a pretty girl
named Vicki Weigle walked up to him with a huge smile on her face.
Ticking, Jeff feared the worst.

Oh god! he thought. *Here comes another person I don't know who's
probably going to say something about my Tourette's.*

Nope.

"Hi, I'm Vicki," she said with a huge smile. "You're Jeff, right?"

"Yeah," Jeff said warily, wondering when she was going to start
making fun of him.

"You just moved to our school, right?"

"Yeah."

"Well, it's great to have you at our school," she said, extending her
hand. "Welcome here!" She handed him a green flyer, then invited him
to Young Life, a Christian youth social organization. "We talk about
scripture and prayer, our relationship with God, and we do a lot of fun
activities," she said. "We even do ice-breaking events for people like you."

That got his attention.

"There's no obligation," she said. "If you'd like to join us there's a
meeting tonight." She smiled again. "If you have any questions about
Young Life, or any questions about teachers or finding your way around
the building, just let me know."

Jeff was shocked. And for the first time he looked a stranger in the eyes and smiled himself. He thanked her and looked at the flyer. "Vicki, I really appreciate this," he said. Then he walked to a pay phone and called his mother.

"Mom," he said. "I just met this really cool girl named Vicki, and she told me about Young Life. And I think I'd like to go."

18

Come on, Jesus. Time to Spill Corn Flakes

RELIGION HAD ALWAYS been confusing for Jeff. Raised in the Catholic church, he believed in God. He *loved* God. It's just that there were times he really wanted to punch him in the nose.

Was God helping him, or torturing him? Did he care about him, or had he forsaken him? If it was possible to be a person who deeply believed in God and deeply *did not* believe in God, Jeff was that person.

His family was very Catholic. His Grandpa Matovic, whom he visited most summers in Greenville, Pennsylvania, had done much of the carpentry work for St. Michael's Catholic Church in that town. When Jeff went to church there he sat between his father and grandfather, often running his hands along the smooth wooden pews thinking *Grandpa made this!*

But as he grew, Jeff's attachment to the church waned. As a boy at St. Bonaventure back in Glenshaw, he went to regular confessions. After his diagnosis, he confessed to fear and confusion regarding the loving God he always heard about in church.

"I'm scared to death," he told the priest at St. Bonnie's. "Father, why is God doing this to me? And with all I'm trying to deal with, why doesn't he help me out a little bit?"

"Jeff," Father Ed replied, "things happen for a reason. And God will watch over you and protect you."

103

Jeff smiled and nodded his head as if he understood.

He didn't.

Did they teach you that line in seminary? he thought. *What a waste of time!*

By the time Jeff became a teenager, he was angry at God. To him, Mass was little more than a stage play filled with empty platitudes. Every week he heard the same two things: Jesus loved him and would walk the hard and lonely road with him. And God had a plan for his life.

God has a plan for my life? he thought. *What's his plan? To ruin it?*

And just where was Jesus when he was suffering? He couldn't help thinking the whole thing was one giant, religious-sounding load of crap.

Still, when he was suffering, he would kneel and pray—for help, for hope, for a miracle. As a teenager Jeff went to church only because his parents insisted. At St. Ladislas Parish in Westlake, Ohio, they sat as close to the front as possible—sometimes in the first row—where Jeff, who couldn't keep still, felt a thousand eyes boring into the back of his skull.

He could just imagine what the parishioners must have thought of the twitchin' teen, the front-row freak, the Sunday spectacle. Too often Mass was fearful, frightening, and embarrassing. He really couldn't get anything out of it because all his energy was directed toward trying to stop the tics. He found that he got more out of praying in the woods or reflecting when running.

Jeff would have done anything not to tic at Mass. He said prayers, counted to a thousand, and took long, deep breaths. It didn't work. One time, as the priest finished the homily by saying "And may God continue to bless you," Jeff's right arm flew out in an uncontrollable jerk, ripping a page out of the mass hymnal in the middle of a dead silence.

Everyone turned to look at Jeff—even the priest.

When everyone sat down, Steve leaned over and whispered, "That was a shitty song. We didn't need that one anyway." Jeff couldn't help but laugh just a little.

Oh, that was it. He was going to hell for sure!

But too many other times it just wasn't funny. Monday mornings, as an eighth grader, he'd wake up and begin to tic before his feet hit the floor. It was winter in Cleveland—cold, gray, and depressing. He *hated* winter. As he'd lie in bed he'd think about the homily the priest had given the day before, and the Jesus who was never there.

The sarcasm came naturally to the smart thirteen-year-old with a body full of pain.

"OK, Jesus," he'd say. "You can come out of the closet now! Time to face the day together, just like you said. *Come on, Jesus!* Time to go spill Corn Flakes on my crisp, white shirt that my OCD made me iron for two hours last night. Then let's go to the bus stop and get made fun of while waiting for the bus. Then let's get on the bus, Jesus. Oh, but we can't sit by the pretty girls. We've got to sit in the back, over the wheel, where we can feel every bump as we tic and twitch all the way to school. But at least I know you'll sit with me, Jesus, cause you *luuuv* me."

Sometimes he questioned God. "Why are you doing this to me?" he'd say out loud. "I'm doing what you tell me to do on Sundays, and I'm doing the best I can. I'm being honest, I feel I'm a giving person, a loving person. *Why do you keep giving me this?* And why do other people have it so easy? Why don't you distribute it a little bit?"

He thought especially about his older brother. While he loved Steve and came to rely on him in so many ways, he also began to resent him and envy all he had. Steve seemed to be God's favorite. He was the golden boy who could do no wrong and had life so easy.

Worse, he seemed to get double blessings from God. Double the love! The double the protection!

Where's mine? Jeff wondered.

Jeff's parents not only understood Jeff's anger at God, they encouraged him to express it. They told him he'd only know if he had a true relationship with the Lord if it changed. Besides, they told him, it was only natural to get angry with God sometimes.

But even they couldn't have known just how angry Jeff was becoming. It wasn't long before they found out.

EXHAUSTED, JEFF BOARDED the bus one day after school, slung his backpack onto a seat, and sat down next to it. This had been the king of crappy days. His tics. The teasing. His teachers. He didn't know what he'd do if one more thing went wrong.

And then it did.

"Hey, dude," a student said in a nerdy voice that sounded like it belonged in a Saturday morning cartoon. "Wanna try somma this?"

Jeff looked up to see an overweight kid with saggy jeans, greasy black hair, and killer BO extending a small, flat, round container. The brown stuff inside was slimy and disgusting—*and it smelled.* Jeff looked at the green tin of Skoal with the kind of pruny face a ten-year-old reserves for a piece of liver. Seething, he backslapped the container out of the boy's hand and then pressed his head against the boy's brow.

"Listen, you asshole," Jeff said. "If you don't get *the fuck* out of my face right now you and your Skoal are going out this bus window. Do you understand me?"

The boy backed up as if Jeff had a gun.

"DO YOU UNDERSTAND ME?"

"Y-yes sir," the boy stammered, his eyes bugging out of his head. "I don't want any trouble. I . . . just want to get off!"

A heavy silence fell as the greasy-haired kid scuttled off the bus. Other students hunched their shoulders and suddenly found something very interesting to look at in their backpacks. On the three-mile ride to Jeff's house no one said a word. Finally home, he threw his book bag on the floor. He heard his mother greet him from the laundry room.

"Hi honey. How are you?"

Jeff steamed past her without a word and stormed into his room. Sometimes he thought it was the only place he could get any peace. The standard-sized ranch-house bedroom had light blue walls and, as a Dallas Cowboys fan, Jeff had persuaded his parents to add a Cowboy-blue stripe around the inside of the room. A full-length mirror hung on the inside of the door. A large wood-grain entertainment center—a birthday gift from his parents—sat against one wall. His stereo system with the dual cassette deck, record player, and radio sat in the middle section, and a twenty-gallon aquarium with colorful fish sat on top. A poster of a red Porsche 944 parked in leaves hung on one wall.

Back in the laundry room Jeff's mother stewed as she finished the last load. You did not throw your book bag down in a heap in Patty Matovic's well-kept house. And you certainly did not disrespect your mother by ignoring her polite greeting.

Minutes later Jeff heard a knock at his door. "May I come in?" his mother said in a stern voice.

He opened the door.

"Did you hear me say hello?" she said.

Jeff put his right hand out as if laying it flat on a table, then made a
chopping motion to cut her off. "Mom," he said. "This is *not* a good time."

Her look softened. She had seen this Jeff before, and she knew in an
instant that this was more serious than simple disrespect. "Why not?"
she said with a soft I-love-you voice.

That's all it took. Jeff's knees went weak as everything seemed to
hit him all at once—everything he had been holding in for so long. He
collapsed onto his bed and bent forward until his head was lying on the
mattress. Then he began to sob. His mother sat down next to him and
wrapped her arm around his back. Jeff reached up with both hands and
put his arms around his mother's neck. As his tears soaked her shirt, he
held on to her with all his strength.

"Aw, honey, just let it out," she said. After a few minutes she left and
returned with an ice-cold washcloth that she placed on his eyes and his
neck. "What happened today?" she asked. "Are you OK? Are you hurt?"

Jeff sat expressionless, staring at his medium blue carpet. Breathing hard, he stared straight ahead before managing to force out a few
words. "I don't know why it has to happen to me, especially all in one
day," he said. "God dammit! I can't take this!"

Carefully, Patty Matovic lifted her son off his bed and supported
him as she walked him down the hallway. "I need to show you something," she said. When they reached the end of the hall she lifted Jeff's
chin and nodded toward a famous poem on the wall that read "Footprints in the Sand."

"This is what you need to know," she said. "And this is all you need
to remember."

The poem told the story of a man who dreamed that his life had
flashed before his eyes as he walked along a beach with God. Sometimes the man saw two sets of footprints. But during his most trying
times he saw only one. "Why haven't you been there for me when I
really needed you?" he asked God.

"The times when you have only seen one set of footprints," the Lord
explained, "is when I carried you."

Jeff knew what it said and didn't care to hear it again. He pulled
away from his mother and walked back to his room. Turning around,
he threw his hands down to his side with a violent karate-chop motion,
and yelled, at the top of his lungs.

"No!" he yelled. "This is *not* the way it is! What that plaque, what that God, and what that church says is *bullshit*!"

"*Jeffrey*!" his mother said.

"No! Everybody in the whole flippin' world has it *so easy* compared to the shit I have to put up with every god damned day! Everybody talks about walking in somebody else's shoes."

And now he was screaming. "I want to put my shoes outside and see if someone would try on my god damned shoes for a change—'cause no one would! The only thing that plaque got wrong is that I am the one doing all the walking, and I've got the whole world on my shoulders! And that's what God needs to know!"

He slammed his door.

Fairly vibrating with anger he stood his extra-long twin mattress against the wall and started beating on it. Short, straight rights and roundhouse lefts. Savage uppercuts that scraped his knuckles and kicks that threatened to rip a hole in the fabric. He whaled on his mattress for several minutes as fast and hard as he could before finally collapsing on the floor out of exhaustion and sleeping until dinner.

— —

BUT NOW EVERYTHING had changed. There was Vicki Weigle, not making fun of him, but smiling at him with kind eyes. There was her green flyer, giving him hope where there was none before.

A Young Life meeting? Young Christians who might be able to see him for who he was on the inside and not prejudge him for what he did on the outside? Yes, he was angry at God. But he remembered what his parents had said about how you knew your relationship was real if it changed. Maybe this was an opportunity for change.

Maybe, he thought, *this was God throwing him a life preserver.*

Why not? he thought. He had avoided people for so long. Jay Blair was a good friend, but he was pretty much all he had. This was his opportunity to make more healthy friendships, get the kind of spiritual guidance he couldn't get in Mass, and get back on track. In a way, he had lost himself after the move. He needed to rebuild the confidence and emotional stability he had in Glenshaw.

That night Jeff went to the meeting. The group read a scripture passage about friendship and loyalty and played an ice-breaking game in which you had to find five people with a name that started with the letter that your name started with. He ticked, but no one made fun of him. And because he felt accepted, he ticked less anyway and let more of his personality show.

Later that year Jeff joined Young Life and even took a two-week trip to Colorado Springs, where he rededicated his life and his service to God and others. He put the letter he wrote about it in his Bible.

Years later he'd look back on the day he met Vicki Weigle as a day that helped change his life and helped him make it through high school. When his mother picked him up from that first meeting, he knew he had found something special.

That night, in the darkness on the ride home, he folded his hands and closed his eyes.

"Thank you," is all he said.

19

Saved by Sports

WHILE FINDING YOUNG Life helped Jeff's spiritual and social life, nothing helped his Tourette's—or his confidence—more than sports. Jeff played on the high school basketball team, ran track, and could fling a football sixty yards in the air. But nowhere was his domination more evident than while running cross-country. Before every race he would step across the starting line and glare back at his competition.

Who thinks they can beat me today? Jeff didn't say the words out loud, but he thought them as he stared down the other runners before moving to the starting line. Some took it as confidence. Others just thought he was cocky.

And what if he was? With his long strides and greyhound-thin body, Jeff dominated cross-country races throughout the high school season. And he wasn't above a little prerace intimidation. But as he paced back and forth there was something none of the other runners knew. He wasn't trying to intimidate them. He had a bigger foe in mind.

As the adrenaline rose in his chest, he fought to hold back an avalanche of tics. When he couldn't, people pointed, called him names, and laughed in his face. He used it all as motivation for this moment.

You know what? he thought as he glared back at the throng of runners edging toward the starting line moments before the race. *None of you have any idea what I have to deal with. None of you! And if I can deal with this, I'm going to destroy you today!*

And then he would. Jeff was built like a racehorse. At six feet five, 175 pounds, with cut, muscular legs that seemed like they were carved from granite, Jeff ran angrily as he blew past competitors to win race after race. He captured all-city honors and had glowing articles written about him in the *Cleveland Plain Dealer.* Each time he wasn't just beating his competition, he was beating his tics, showing them who was boss.

Fittingly, his success in cross-country brought in scholarship offers from across the country. In his junior year he received dozens of letters from top colleges that wanted him to run for them, including prestigious schools such as Arizona State and the University of North Carolina.

From the time he was a boy, sports had leveled the playing field that Tourette's had tilted. Sports came easy. In grade school kickball games he'd kick the ball so far it would get lost in the woods. He was so dominant in dodgeball his friends dubbed him "the Weltmaster," and his gym teacher banned him from playing. For some, Jeff's prowess at sports never made sense. Didn't he have a *movement* disorder? How could he focus his twitching muscles enough to be that good?

Actually, it made perfect sense. Tourette's is not an inability to move but the constant *desire* to move. Moving was not the problem, staying still was. Sports was Jeff's way to escape and excel. Most of the time the motion satisfied his urge to move, and the intense concentration focused his muscles and calmed his tics.

Most of the time. He still ticked during some sports.

Take basketball. Jeff's parents remember one game where they watched him twitch at the free throw line for what seemed like several minutes before he could shoot. One time at basketball practice during his freshman year at Bay Village High School, a teammate named Ben, who liked to tease Jeff, had the ball at the top of the key. Suddenly he fired a hard chest pass Jeff's way. Jeff didn't see it because he was ticking. The ball bounced off his chest and rolled away.

"Sorry, Matovic," Ben said with a sneer. "I hit you right in the numbers. I'll try to make the pass better the next time."

Another time the coach asked Jeff to set a pick, which means to run to a spot on the court and—while standing still—block the path of a defender so one of his teammates can get an open shot. Jeff ran to the spot, but as he tried to set the pick he could not stand still. His convulsions made it look like he pushed the defender instead, which is a foul.

"Come on, spaz boy! Get it right," said Ben. "We've only gone over this a hundred times now. Quit shaking and doing all your crazy stuff so we can get out of here!"

But sometimes his tics actually came in handy. In the sixth grade Jeff's friend Kevin stole the ball and keyed a two-on-one fast break in a tense night game against crosstown rival St. Teresa's. With the score tied in the second half, Jeff was running on the right wing as Kevin fed him a bounce pass at the foul line. Jeff took the ball and streaked toward the hoop just ahead of a backpedaling player hustling to block his driving layup. But when he arrived at the basket, Jeff's Tourette's suddenly made him stop and tic before going up for the shot. He gripped the ball with his large hands like a vise as if throwing a chest pass and screamed "Huh! Huh!" as loudly as he could. His arms shot out wildly toward the St. Teresa cheerleaders. He didn't throw the ball at them, but his exaggerated motions convinced them that he might. Frightened, they scattered, bumped into one another, and threw their pompons into the air. By the time he went up for the shot, the defender—unable to stop his momentum—landed on Jeff's back as he made the shot. The referee called the other player for a foul. Jeff made the foul shot to complete the three-point play and help his team win the game.

"Hey, Jeff," Kevin said, "you'll have to teach me that move someday. That was awesome!"

But most of the time Jeff's tics were not a factor in the sports he played. And most of the time—tics or no tics—he dominated. Especially when he got to run.

In the spring of 1990, during the district meet in the Cleveland suburb of Olmstead Falls, Jeff's coach came to him with a request after a Bay Village runner got injured.

"Little switch in plans," his coach said. "We don't have four for the four-by-four [mile] relay. I need you to jump in there."

Already fatigued after running the half mile and the mile and just finishing the four-mile relay twenty minutes earlier, Jeff nodded his head. "No problem, coach," he said. "You can rely on me. When is it?"

"It starts in about four minutes," he said. "Go warm up."

There were seven schools in the meet, but by this time only two—Westlake and Bay Village—were still alive to win the district title. Jeff had run the 400 before, but he certainly didn't specialize in it. His coach expected him to run the final lap in the race—the all-important anchor leg. It had all come down to this race, which would determine the district champion.

When the gun went off, Jeff forgot about his fatigue. During the first leg, Bay Village fell a little behind, then the second racer pulled even. As the other runners finished their legs, Jeff checked out his competition and jumped up and down on the track to keep loose. By the time he got the baton, the Westlake runner had about a five-second lead. The Olmstead runner was even farther in front. He kicked quickly into top gear.

"Turn and burn!" Jeff screamed, quoting a line from the movie *Top Gun*. He forgot strategy, forgot saving his "kick" for the end. He ran like a man possessed, full out, as fast as he could go. If he wanted the title, he had to pass those runners, and it was going to take everything he had.

At the 300-meter mark Jeff had pulled to within 10 meters of the Westlake runner. The Olmstead Falls runner was still another five meters in front. But Jeff was gaining on them—fast. He gulped air and dug deep.

A hundred meters for the title, he thought. He reached back and asked his body for more. He knew he was going to break his own record. But how much would he have left at the end?

Everything hurt. His lungs burned. He thought about all the times Tourette's had limited him and stopped him from doing the things he wanted. *Not this time*, he thought. He ran as fast as he could.

And then he ran faster. "This is *my* one hundred," he said. "You're not taking this from me." With twenty meters left to the finish line, he blew past the Westlake runner and then, with a final lean, nipped the Olmstead Falls runner at the wire. Ecstatic, Jeff raised the baton in the air.

"Now that's how we do that!" he yelled, as he fired the baton hard against a fence.

A scream went up from the Bay Village team. Everyone stood and ran toward him after he fell down from exhaustion in the grassy infield. He wore a broad smile as his teammates piled on top of him, dousing him with water and Gatorade while yelling "Champs! Champs! Champs!" Jeff had shaken off his fatigue to run the anchor leg in 49.8 seconds, his personal best.

After getting up, he saw his father in the stands. Jim Matovic looked at his watch and shrugged as if to say, "I don't know how you did that."

Jeff loved to run. When his tics became unbearable he would run around the block. It wasn't a jog, it was a full sprint designed to release stress, pain, and anger. When he was done he'd take a moment to catch his breath, and then do it again.

"You know what?" he'd say to his Tourette's. "I still have more. And I'm going to beat you! I'm going to beat you down to the ground!"

As he ran he would talk to his tics, cursing and calling them vile names that would have shocked his parents. The sprinting did double duty. While it exhausted him, it also sapped the power from his tics. And in a way it empowered him to think that he could handle anything his tics could throw at him.

His running paid dividends in other ways as well. As a senior he qualified for the state championships hosted at Ohio State University by running a 4:24 in the mile. His father went with him to watch, and even took a lap with him around the Ohio State track.

While he was the best at running, Jeff excelled in all sports. He could throw a baseball so hard it would leave seam impressions in a catcher's mitt. And as good as he was at baseball, he was even better at football.

One fall day while waiting for his cross-country coach on the track, he finished his stretching and then grabbed a football to play catch with one of his teammates, Bryan Putnam. Jeff pretended to take a snap from center.

"Putnam goes deep," he said as he took a three-step drop and launched a fifty-five-yard bomb that hit his friend in stride.

Nearby he heard the grunts and hard hits of football practice. After a while Coach Kaiser, the varsity football coach who also coached Jeff in track in the spring, noticed the power and precision in Jeff's tight spirals. After making the lineman run wind sprints, he walked over to greet him. "So what are your goals for cross-country this season?" he asked.

"I'm looking to take my team to the state meet in Columbus again, and place individually as an All-Ohioan," Jeff said.

The coach nodded, then looked Jeff squarely in the eye. "I saw you throwing that football around," he said. "Why haven't you tried out for the football team?"

"I don't know," Jeff said. "I guess it's because I've never played organized football and I'd be way behind the learning curve."

The coach leaned in closer. "How would you like to skip cross-country and be my starting quarterback?" he said. "I'll get you up to speed on the playbook after and before school. And with your grades, I know you're a smart guy, so the learning process won't be that hard for you. Whaddaya say?"

"I don't know, Coach," a shocked Jeff said. "I've already committed to my team in cross-country, and I'm involved in so many other things, including hoops in the winter and track in the spring."

Just then, Denny Sheppard, the cross-country coach, grabbed Jeff by the arm and pulled him aside. He glared at Coach Kaiser with a hint of a smile. "You're not getting my star runner to play on that field," he said. "I've already recruited him."

— —

I LOVED HEARING about Jeff's passion for sports. I understood exactly how they made him feel, because they made me feel the same way.

Sports were my refuge too. In many ways my life was defined by sports. I always felt better when I was moving. I played baseball, basketball, football, racquetball, and golf. I batted tennis balls against the walls of my house and threw SuperBalls against the walls of my school. I played catch with my friends and with my father. Growing up in the 1960s, I won the Presidential Physical Fitness Award every year I was eligible. It was a big deal back then and a great source of pride. This was a time in America when awards still meant something. They weren't given out like cups of water. The standards were high, and you had to earn it. And when you did you could be justifiably proud of yourself—and I was.

I don't mean to brag, but with no false modesty, I was an exceptional athlete. People could mock me, tease me, laugh at me, point at me, call me names, or make jokes behind my back. But when it came to picking teams for a sport, they knew they'd better pick me high, or I would make them pay. For a small guy—five feet nine and a half—I once recorded a forty-inch vertical jump. I could dunk volleyballs and block the shots of people half a foot taller than me. In football I was so quick that often no one on the other team could touch me, let alone catch me. I would dart and juke my way through crowds again and again to score multiple touchdowns.

I never seriously went out for football because of my Tourette's. I simply hated to have anything on my head, and couldn't concentrate on anything else.

In high school I did 250 sit-ups a night. It gave me rock-hard abdominal muscles and even helped improve my self-esteem. One day a classmate heard me talking about the tightness of my stomach.

"If your stomach's so tough, why don't you let me hit you as hard as I can?" he asked.

"OK," I said, tightening my stomach and putting my hands on my hips. "Go ahead." The teacher was late that day, and the whole class watched. The intensity of the situation helped me focus and temporarily blocked my tics. The guy who hit me was much larger than I was. He reared back with his right arm and hit me dead in the middle of my stomach with a savage punch.

Thwwack!

His large fist bounced off my powerful stomach muscles. I didn't move or react. An "Ooohh" purred through the classroom.

"OK," I said. "Now let me hit you."

When he refused I gained an important measure of respect—both from my classmates and from myself. I might have been the weird kid who shook his head. But I was also the amazing athlete with the rock-hard abs. Like Jeff, success in sports saved me and gave me the confidence to conquer other challenges in my life—like college.

After graduating from high school in 1976, I enrolled in the University of Nebraska, the school where most of my friends were going. And Jeff? While he could have attended many schools out of state, in 1991 he chose John Carroll University, a Jesuit school in the Cleveland suburb of University Heights. With his Tourette's as the wild card, it was critical to remain close to home, and Carroll was only forty-five minutes away from his parents' house. Besides, the college offered him scholarships, his father had gone there, and it was an excellent school. In an effort to better understand himself, he majored in psychology. There was only one problem: his Tourette's. As he grew older, it grew stronger. And unfortunately John Carroll didn't offer a class in surviving intractable pain.

That he'd have to learn on his own.

20

"God Bless You, Jeff Foxworthy!"

STAGGERING IN THE middle of his dorm room, Jeff grimaced and then doubled over in pain. It was hard to think, and even harder to breathe.

This was bad. It felt as if Hulk Hogan had him in a leg lock and was crushing him like a walnut. But it wasn't just the pain. For five agonizing minutes he had ridden out a brutal explosion of tics. These were no ordinary twitches—they were sustained and powerful jerks, the kind of dangerous tics that could fling you around a room like you were *nothing*. Unable to stop the lurching spasms, he banged his knuckles, bruised his shins, and sliced open his forearm on the sharp corner of a wooden dresser. As he desperately sought to protect himself against more serious injury, he reached out with his long arms and hugged the base of his wooden desk.

But even that couldn't keep him anchored. He had become his own earthquake. As violent full-body tremors sent him stumbling through the room, they took the desk with him. Items flew off the desktop and skittered across the tile floor—ballpoint pens, a John Carroll coffee mug, his wallet and keys. Heavy textbooks slid off the edge and thumped him on the side of the head.

"Please, God," he cried.

Losing his grip on the desk, he tried to stand. He wobbled like a drunk before another explosive tic threw him hard onto a multicolored area rug. Too tired to get back up, he lay in a pool of his own sweat and flopped on the floor like a 170-pound fish out of water. Bouncing high off the ground, he repeatedly smashed his head and his tailbone onto the floor. The only thing worse was when the bounces flipped him over and he began slamming his face into the floor.

Horrible thoughts flooded through his bruised brain. What the hell was he doing in college? *I suck at this!* he told himself. *I should quit. My grades aren't good enough, and I'll never make it four years. Besides, look at me. I'm a freak!*

He dreamed of going to the train station and buying a ticket to anywhere, just to escape the pressure. But he couldn't do that. He'd worked too hard to get here. He'd have to find a way to survive.

Usually he played loud music to calm himself down. It would have been more polite to use headphones so he wouldn't bother the other students, but he couldn't. They were way too hot. Besides, they'd never stay on his head. So he cranked up the music from large floor speakers. It wasn't a problem during the day.

But in the middle of the night . . .

"Matovic!" a student screamed from down the hall. "Would you shut that shit off! It's three in the morning, and I've got an exam in five hours! Jesus!"

"Sorry, man," Jeff would yell. "You know what I have to deal with." But when his tics got *really* bad, when they started throwing him around the room like this, not even music could help.

He knew what he had to do. Summoning what little strength he had left, he rose to one knee and managed to push the start button on his five-disc CD player. He lay spread-eagle on the ground as he closed his eyes, took a big breath, and let a familiar voice wash over him in its unmistakable high-pitched Southern drawl.

> Everywhere you go in Georgia now, all they talk about is the Olympics coming there in '96. And my whole thought is—"The Olympics in Georgia: God, you know we're goin' screw that up!"
> I guarantee ya, when they let those doves go in the opening ceremony there are going to be guys in the parking lot with shotguns. (Boom! Boom! Boom!)
>
> "Hey Ed! I got a whiiiite one!"

At John Carroll the best medicine Jeff had to help him survive his severe tics didn't come from a prescription bottle; it came from a home-spun Southerner who would go on to become the bestselling comedy recording artist of all time. The comedy of Jeff Foxworthy not only made Jeff laugh, it also helped save his life.

> Hell, the Olympic rings will be five old tires nailed together. 'Cause they burn a looonnng time. I'm going back to see this. I mean, if nothing else, the opening ceremony.
>
> "GREE-TINGS, Y'ALL! AND WELCOME ALL YOU DANG FOREIGNERS FROM OTHER NATIONS. DEAR LORD, BE WITH OUR GUESTS AND PREPARE THEM FOR THE BUTT WHIPPING THEY ARE ABOUT TO RECEIVE!"

Jeff laughed as he wiped the blood from his arm and repeated the words verbatim. Every inch of his body hurt.

Laughing felt good. It gave him something to focus on, made him feel human again, and returned badly needed energy to his body. He always considered the play button on his CD player a *healing* button—because that's exactly what Jeff Foxworthy's humor did for him.

> In a lot of parts of the country people hear me talk, they automati-cally want to deduct a hundred IQ points. 'Cause apparently the Southern accent is not the most "intelligent-sounding" accent. And to be honest, none of us would like to hear our brain surgeon say: "Arright, now what we goin' do is . . . saw the top of your head off, root around in there with a stick, and see if we can't find that dadburned clot." People are like, "No thanks. I'll just die."

Somehow Foxworthy's pithy observations about life rebooted Jeff's system. They not only calmed his body, but also balanced his mind, helping him to come back from bad places and see things in a more healthy perspective. He owned three of Jeff Foxworthy's CDs, and he never took them out of his CD player. He knew that at some point, if his tics grew bad enough, he would listen to them again.

> If I'm around my family for more than a week, I start having fantasies that maybe I'm adopted and have a normal family that's desperately trying to find me. But you know what? You don't have

the stupidest family in the world. You don't have the goofiest family in the world. And if you ever need to verify that, all you have to do is go to a state fair. Five minutes at a fair, you'll be going, "You know what? We're all right. We're dang near royalty!"

After several minutes, Jeff felt good enough to get up, get himself a drink of water, put a wet washcloth over his head, and climb in bed. He knew each of the bits by heart. Like Bill Cosby, another of his favorites, Foxworthy talked about universal experiences. After a few more minutes Jeff was bouncing on the mattress.

Cool, he thought. *I'm bouncing on my mattress, but I'm doing it like a normal person!*

You ever see people so ugly you have to get somebody else to verify it? "Come 'ere, y'all gotta see this man! Get outta line. It's worth it! Over by the cotton candy. Don't look. Don't look. Don't look. Is that the hairiest back you've ever seen? Looks like Big Foot in a tank top. OH GOD, IT'S A WO–MAN! And she's got kids. Somebody slept with that WO–MANNNN!"

Jeff smiled as he screamed the word "WO–MANN!" right along with Foxworthy. The relief it brought him was real and immediate.

Foxworthy's humor helped Jeff in other ways too. Since he didn't have to worry about ticking as long as his comedy CDs were playing, he was able to meet new people over Foxworthy listening sessions. The comedy helped him break the ice, make friends—even get a girlfriend. But most of all it gave him peace and assured him that no matter how bad things got, there was always something that could make him smile and help him recover.

If your wife has ever said, "Come move this transmission so I can take a bath"—you might be a redneck. If you've ever been accused of lying through your tooth . . . If you think "The Nutcracker" is something you did off the high dive . . . If somebody hollers "Hoedown" and your girlfriend hits the floor . . .

Laughing so hard he started to cry, Jeff wiped a tear from his eye. His body finally calm, he inhaled a deep, peaceful breath and uttered a familiar, five-word prayer.

"God bless you, Jeff Foxworthy."

21

John Carroll University

A SINGLE PRAYER book sat open on a tiny table, a silent sentry in a small chapel at Cleveland's John Carroll University. The late-evening darkness made the lights inside seem even brighter. A golden crucifix graced the wall of the gleaming cherry altar.

Alone in the room, Jeff melted into his favorite cushioned chair— the second chair in the second row. His long arms relaxed until they turned to rubber and started to tingle. He did deep breathing exercises and progressive muscle relaxation. As he reclined he rested his head against the back of the chair and let the quiet of the room bake into him like the sun.

Jeff was a regular here. Open day and night, St. Francis Chapel served as both a safe haven and a refueling station. For Jeff it was just like the comedy of Jeff Foxworthy. He didn't think he could go on without it.

Breathing deeply, he closed his eyes and tried to relax. As he did he prayed out loud.

"St. Michael the Archangel, defend us in battle. Be our safe-guard against the wickedness and snares of the devil. May God rebuke him, we humbly pray, and do thou, oh Prince of the Heavenly Hosts, by the Power of God, cast down into hell Satan, and all his evil spirits who wander now throughout the world seeking the ruin of souls. Amen."

Later he directed his prayers to the Virgin Mary. And to Jesus. And directly to God. "Take this burden," he said in a small voice, cracking with emotion. "Lift my spirits. . . . Give me the strength to go on."

If there was one thing Jeff had learned, it was how to go on. One more minute. One more hour. One more day. The pain couldn't defeat him if he didn't let it.

After fifteen minutes he had spoken his piece and relaxed as much as his body would allow. He got up and headed for the door. Before leaving, he stopped to sign the prayer book on the tiny table. He always signed it the same way: "Your disciple—J." And he kept the prayer book open so he could envision his prayers being soaked up while he was away.

⤙ ⤚

JEFF TOLD ME the story about his time praying at St. Francis Chapel during one of our interviews about his college years. I loved that story, and the way he told it. When he talked about St. Francis chapel he got this indescribable look on his face, and I felt like I was there with him in a place of peace.

I had my special places too—places I would go to pray or be alone during college. One of them was in the stacks in the basement of Love Library at the University of Nebraska. It was cool and dark, and the small cubicles were hidden away in an industrial area that time had forgotten. There was a certain privacy, and serenity, to the area that I always loved.

During college I got a job cleaning our church, Southminster United Methodist. I had a key and often worked nights when no one was there. My favorite place was the balcony, overlooking the gleaming pews and stained glass windows. It was so peaceful up there. And beautiful. I remember many nights after finishing my work I'd go up to the balcony and talk to God. Kneeling at the opened window in the echoing silence, a feeling of peace and love surrounded me. My prayers were silent and from my heart, and when I was there I felt safe and like nothing could hurt me—not even my tics.

I imagine that's what Jeff felt like at St. Francis Chapel.

⤙ ⤚

IN THE SUMMER of 2008 I actually got to sit in St. Francis Chapel. On one of my visits to Cleveland, Jeff took me there. I can't describe it, but I felt a special connection there with Jeff. It was as if in that room his pain and my pain, his life and my life, had come together in a new way. In my mind I could see him in that chair, hurting and ticking and praying for solace. I wished so much I could have been there to tell him to fight on, to *hang* on, and how brave I thought he was just for being there in the first place.

To this day I don't think people realize what kind of strength it took to look that kind of pain in the face and refuse to give in. What he did was extraordinary, and I don't think another person in a hundred could have done it.

College was worse for him than high school. A lot worse. A psychology major, Jeff studied hard. But as his tics strengthened and his medications could no longer control them as well as they once did, he worried he might not be able to graduate, let alone maintain the 3.0 grade-point average required to keep his scholarships. Some days were so bad he openly wished for death so the pain would stop.

Through the help of his advisor, Dr. Helen Murphy, he got help in the form of untimed tests and special rooms where he could take final exams by himself. He also got the kind of personal support and friendship that helped him cope.

— —

I TOOK A second trip to Cleveland. After talking to Jeff for what seemed like hundreds of hours on the phone, I felt it was important to look him in the eyes as I heard his stories. I also wanted to get to know his wife, Debra, better, because without her strength, he wouldn't have been around to tell anybody anything.

Deb is one of a kind—fiery, determined, stubborn, and sweet, a smallish whirlwind of a woman with dark hair with reddish highlights who is fiercely protective of the family she loves. She is the silent hero of that family, and I wanted her to know that she meant every bit as much to me as Jeff.

Jeff and Deb invited me to stay at their two-story house in the Cleveland suburb of South Euclid. I had a late flight and worried about my ride as a delay pushed my arrival to well after midnight. But when

I deplaned at Hopkins International Airport, there was Jeff beaming from ear to ear.

My trip to Cleveland was filled with wonderful experiences. I got to know Jeff and Deb's teenagers, Bonnie and Mike, and meet a few of their friends. I ate with Jeff and his family and with Deb and her family. Jeff and I even stayed up late one night and watched one of his favorite movies. While *Rocky IV* isn't what you'd call high art, Jeff loved it for other reasons. He identified with Rocky, who defied the odds by using willpower to outwork and overcome a steroid-fueled killing machine named Ivan Drago. Jeff saw himself as Rocky, and his Tourette's as Drago. We watched the movie after midnight in the living room. We cheered so loudly we woke up Deb, who walked down the stairs in her robe to ask us to pipe down.

As fun as the movie was, I hadn't come for that. What I really needed to do was continue our interviews. The next morning Jeff and I decided to talk at John Carroll University. I was excited. I had heard the stories—now I wanted to see where they happened.

For Jeff, college was something to survive as much as experience. But in a weird way, the difficulty of his courses helped him to focus. Of course, other students asked about his strange movements. But being a psychology major, he took most of his classes with other psych majors and pre-med students. When he explained, they understood. His teachers understood his condition as well, making accommodations for him when necessary.

For fun, Jeff played Nintendo in his dorm room with other residents. He let them know about his tics, and they accepted him. He and friends often dressed up and went downtown to the dance clubs. Jeff *loved* going to the clubs. With the loud music, the dancing, the darkness, and the fact that many of the people there were drunk, he could tic all he wanted and nobody ever noticed.

Jeff didn't drink or do drugs in college. Not only did he not think it was the right thing to do, he didn't want to risk drug interactions with his medications. Plus, as an athlete, he valued his body too much to mess it up.

One of Jeff's best stories concerned the time he kicked his roommate, Paul Knaus, as Paul walked in the door of their tiny dorm room. Jeff was relaxing on the lower part of their bunk bed, trying to get his tics to calm down—not so easy in the August heat. The doorway was inches away from Jeff's large feet, which hung off the end of the mattress. Suddenly Paul walked through the door carrying two plastic grocery bags. His appearance startled Jeff and fueled a violent leg tic that blasted Paul in the right kidney, causing groceries to fly everywhere and Paul to crash into the door frame and crumple to the tile floor.

"Ohhhh!" Paul screamed.

"Oh, Christ!" Jeff said. "I didn't mean it! It was my tics!"

Paul writhed in pain in a fetal position, next to a broken jar of Prego spaghetti sauce. Short of breath and barely able to talk, he slowly rolled onto his back.

"Been . . . one of those days for you, huh?" he said through a painful smile.

— ◆ —

THE CAMPUS OF John Carroll was as clean as it was beautiful. Sidewalks snaked through well-manicured grass dotted with large trees, classy red brick buildings, and statues of educators and saints.

"That was my dorm room right there," Jeff said, pointing to a large, red brick building.

"Post-it Notes," I said, referencing a different story.

"Yeah," he said, "I'll never forget that day."

During his junior year, Jeff and Paul had a large project on gun control for their debate class. They had the pro, or affirmative, position in a Lincoln-Douglas style debate. They researched the topic and meticulously organized their best points with pink, purple, and green Post-it Notes that they stuck on two walls of their dorm room, outlining a flowchart of their arguments. Jeff loved the Post-it Notes, or at least his OCD did. They were perfectly spaced and completely even. He knew how many there were. He cataloged the colors and counted them over and over in his mind.

Later, when Jeff and Paul were talking to friends in the hall, another resident removed the Post-its and scattered them on the floor as a joke. When Jeff saw the prank he became livid.

"What the hell did you do?" he yelled at the prankster.

This was not good. He expected the Post-it Notes to be on the wall, perfectly spaced and completely even. He wanted to catalog them and count them over and over in his mind. Now he couldn't. He felt the panic to his bones. He had to pick them up and put them back exactly where they were. But there were so many of them. And he couldn't figure out where they went.

"This is so uncool," he said to the student who took them down. "If you ever do this again, so help me God I will wake you at three in the morning saying your car's on fire!"

Anxiety began roiling inside him. He began to panic, which supercharged his Tourette's. The tension was off the charts. He had to release it, or he didn't know what would happen!

He grabbed his basketball. "Paul," he said, breathing hard and trying unsuccessfully to hold back the powerful spasms. "I'll be back in a few hours. If I'm not back in three, come get me. I'll be at the gym."

With that he ran outside into the blackness. He knew the gym wouldn't be open that late. But he had to try. At the gym he ran into a janitor.

"You know what," he said, nervously pounding on the basketball. "If you don't let me in I'm going to go *crazy*!"

"You must really love this sport," the confused janitor said. "But you know I can't let you in with security and all," he said.

"Forget security!" Jeff yelled, fairly vibrating with a type of powerful, unbearable insanity. "Let me into this gym—*right now*!" Taken aback, the stunned janitor opened the door.

This was a Tourette's emergency. Running furiously, Jeff dribbled and shot for three hours. It was a long shot, but if he could focus his mind and his body while expending maximum energy he just might be able to rob the tics of their power through sheer exhaustion. Dribble by dribble, it worked.

Back in the dorm room, Paul worked for two and a half hours to put the Post-it Notes back up. But this time he taped them permanently to a couple pieces of poster board that they could fold up and put away.

I looked at Jeff with curious eyes.

"What?"

"Well, you showed me where the Post-it Note story happened. Are you going to show me where the Vanilla Thunder story happened too?"

He smiled. "That's where I was going next."

We walked until we got to the Don Shula Sports Arena, where John Carroll played its college basketball games. We sat in the upper seats to get a better perspective on the floor while Jeff recounted the story of how in his freshman year he had been given the nickname "Vanilla Thunder."

To kick off the season, the school planned an all-school celebration in the gym at midnight featuring the members of the basketball team performing skits. One of the highlights of the celebration that year was a dunk contest featuring five students, including Jeff, who had tried out and earned a spot. Shortly before midnight on the night of the big rally, Jeff warmed up on the floor of the gym as the band played fight songs and students got ready for the party.

"Hey, Matovic," yelled one of the John Carroll players, "show me what you got."

Finally, Jeff thought. Here was a chance to prove that he was more than some spaz who twitched like a puppet on a string. *Show you what I got?* he thought. *Damn right.* The lanky right-hander eyed the basket and tossed the ball underhanded high off the left side of the glass backboard as he sprinted toward the basket. He leapt high in the air and reached his right hand far behind him to cup the ball. He twisted his body in the air and eyed the rim for a windmill dunk.

It would have been perfect if it hadn't been for one thing. Because of his battles with his tics, Jeff had a force inside of him greater than anyone knew, a force borne of determination, frustration, and raw, naked anger. When he slammed the ball through the hoop he was symbolically striking back against years of pain and embarrassment. Unfortunately, his years of pent-up rage were a little more than the hoop could handle. With a loud crack, the backboard exploded into a thousand pieces as if it had been blasted with a shotgun. When Jeff landed on the court, rim in hand, thousands of pieces of shattered backboard rained on him like a Plexiglas shower.

The crowd exploded. Seconds later Jeff heard Paul shouting from the upper level. "Oh, *hell yes! Hell yes!* That's my *boy!*"

Mortified, Jeff looked around to see if he was in trouble. But all he could see was the crowd, exploding in cheers and spilling onto the court to grab pieces of the shattered backboard and stuff them in their pockets as souvenirs. He hadn't meant to break the backboard. But since he had, for one shining moment he was the coolest guy on campus.

The evening's celebration had to be postponed several days until the backboard could be replaced. The event even made it into a brief on the sports page of the *Cleveland Plain Dealer.*

Jeff's backboard-shattering dunk recalled similar feats by Darryl Dawkins, a large and intimidating dunking machine who played for the Philadelphia 76ers. Dawkins was affectionately nicknamed Chocolate Thunder. After Jeff broke John Carroll's backboard, friends dubbed him Vanilla Thunder.

IT WASN'T EASY, but Jeff finished his four years at John Carroll. For Jeff, graduating from college with a degree in psychology felt like slaying a giant with a slingshot. In cap and gown he had defeated his Tourette's and done something none of the experts thought possible.

Graduation was a reverent occasion. Before the graduates walked across the stage, the president of the university requested that audience members hold their applause until all students had been announced.

Right.

Jeff beamed as he walked across the stage. Just before he reached for his diploma, a lone voice sliced through the silence and echoed through the quad.

"Way to go, Jeff!" his brother Steve yelled.

Jeff smiled. The crowd began to clap. Later, in a moment his mother captured in a photo, his father closed his eyes and enfolded his youngest son in a warm embrace after the graduation ceremony.

"Dad," Jeff whispered. "This is as much for you as it is for me."

22

Deep Brain Stimulation

BRAIN CELLS, CALLED neurons, communicate with one another through a series of electrical impulses. In a properly functioning brain this electrical communication is in harmony, like a well-conducted orchestra. In brains with movement disorders that orchestra may be out of tune or off-tempo. Deep brain stimulation (DBS) may affect the tune and tempo, though doctors don't quite know why or how. In DBS, a battery implanted in the chest delivers steady pulses of electricity to a targeted area of the brain. The current alters dysfunctional electrical activity in that area. Specialists adjust the speed, strength, and length of the electrical pulses in an attempt to produce a desired result. Accepted as a way of quelling tremors that can afflict people with Parkinson's disease, dystonia, and essential tremor, DBS has shown promise for improving other ailments, including chronic pain and depression.

———

AFTER COLLEGE, JEFF took a series of jobs—including one in Boston working with autistic children—that never seemed to work out. As he fought his tics, he suffered setbacks and bouts with depression. When he returned to Cleveland, he just wanted to find a way to be happy. He began dating a woman named Maxine. She was kind and treated him nicely. Maybe that was what would make him happy.

They married in 1998. But they were very young and they didn't know each other as well as they should have. Despite their best efforts, the marriage failed. Several years later, they had it annulled. But while she ultimately wasn't right for Jeff, Maxine cared greatly for him and helped start the research that ultimately led him to the operating table.

Another person who helped was a man named Ed Cwalinski. Jeff had never heard that name until he watched an episode of ABC's *20/20* in August 2001. But after he heard it, he couldn't get it out of his head. Soon there was something else he couldn't get out of his head—the possibility that deep brain stimulation, or DBS, could get rid of his tics.

The *20/20* story showed how Cwalinski had undergone the operation to treat a severe case of dystonia that had curved his spine into the shape of the letter *C*. After researching the surgery on the Internet, Jeff found that DBS was approved for several movement disorders but not for Tourette's. Jeff didn't see why it couldn't be. It made sense. Dystonia was a movement disorder and so was Tourette's. Why couldn't DBS be the answer he was looking for?

From 2001 through January 2003, the surgery became Jeff's greatest obsession—and his greatest hope. He requested information by mail and over the phone from the National Institutes of Health, Johns Hopkins, and mental health institutions throughout the world. While he didn't get many returned calls, he did receive a lot of mail—boxes full—explaining the operation. He also researched his own condition further as he continued searching for a way to connect DBS to Tourette Syndrome. There didn't seem to be any.

All you need is one, he told himself. *Keep looking!*

For Jeff, trying to search the Internet while dozens of powerful tics wrenched his body this way and that was like trying to play the piano on a bucking bronco. Worse, when his fingers hit the wrong keys, it could send him to some "interesting" places. Once Google took him to a "big and busty" porn site, where an unattractive older woman with enormous, exposed breasts was smiling back at him in a trashy sort of way.

"Oh, God, no," Jeff said. "I don't want to see that!"

Sometimes Jeff would call his parents to tell them what interesting new sites he had landed on with his tics. He told them about the porn site.

"Oh, Jeff, that's *nasty*!" his mother said.

Then, following a silence, his father said, "What's that address again? I've got a pencil."

"Jim!" he heard his mother say.

Jeff did his research in the bedroom of a small apartment on the third floor of a large, white apartment building in the Cleveland suburb of Brooklyn, Ohio. Several boxes sat on the floor. On the outside of two boxes he had written MAIL SENT and MAIL RECEIVED. Another box was marked INTERNET RESEARCH and contained more than fifty manila folders on research pertaining to DBS, doctors who performed it around the world, his own condition, and possible links. That box was so packed with files he actually had to duct tape it in two different places because it was bursting at the seams. He also had another box labeled CALL BACK INFO FROM DOCTORS/CONTACTS. That was the one box he wished were full.

It was virtually empty.

He sat in a small bedroom at a light-colored wooden desk, staring at his Compaq PC. To the right sat a black desk lamp and a blue John Carroll coffee mug filled with pens and highlighters. In front of the mug a notebook tracked his research. Along the border of his monitor were printed quotations. One read "GOING AROUND IT, OVER IT, OR THROUGH IT"—WALTER PAYTON. On the left side of his monitor he had taped a photocopied picture from the DVD case of the movie *Rocky IV.* It was a picture of the scene, in round two, where Rocky had cut Ivan Drago, the nearly invincible Russian fighter.

He kept a hand towel on the right hand side of the desk that he often chilled in the freezer to cool himself off after prolonged ticking heated him up. Sometimes he would freeze a beach towel and drape it over the back of his chair. Most times he sat at the desk in basketball shorts with no shirt. Two fans—an oscillating fan on his desk and a large, square floor fan—blew air directly on him.

One of the things he treasured the most was an enlarged prayer card of St. Dymphna, the patron saint of mental diseases, hanging on his wall to the right of his desk. Many nights he prayed to St. Dymphna that DBS might be his answer. But first he'd have to find out whether he was even a candidate for the surgery. That information was difficult to find. Finally he found a site from a major US hospital that confirmed that—at least according to his symptoms and his history—he could be. He began calling hospital neurology departments directly, asking to speak to surgeons about the possibility of performing the operation on him. He tried not to get discouraged. But it was hard. Over and over the answer was the same: "We don't do deep brain stimulation for Tourette's."

23

Cemetery Man

JEFF AND I talked for hours at John Carroll. More important, we bonded. After shooting hoops at the gym and getting some lunch, Jeff took me to see an award the school had given him for courage. Turns out the Campion Shield for Heroism award had only been given twice before in the hundred-year history of the school. I took a picture of it in its glass case.

"Impressive!" I said. "You're a friggin' hero, man."

Jeff posed proudly, chest out, as if he were a superhero. I swung my camera around and pretended to take a shot before dropping it to my side.

"You wish," I said. "But seriously. That is *very* cool."

At the library we resumed our interview. He shared with me, and I with him, personal details of our lives and our struggles that we had never told anyone else. We cried together, and for the first time he called me "brother."

Most of our interview was happy, but I knew rough patches lay ahead. Jeff pulled out a journal and read intensely personal poems he had written in the depths of despair. They talked about death, betrayal, and expressed anger in vile and vulgar ways. Many of the bitter and hate-filled musings were intensely shocking and out of character for the Jeff I knew, and they made me uncomfortable. We knew we could have included the worst of them in this book for shock value. But that wouldn't have been right. Tame by comparison, this one gives but a small glimpse into the confusion, anger, and pain that Tourette's can cause.

Directionless and Powerless by a Man Named Jeffrey Paul Matovic, Unknown to Himself

I don't want to feel anymore. I don't want to hear the constant noise inside my head. I don't want to feel lost anymore. I don't want to feel anything. I feel so mixed up. I am so lost in a world that I don't understand.

Why can't I know myself? Why can't I just be me? Hell is on the earth right now as I live in a confused, directionless, ever changing body. Hell is the voice in my head that shouts all the time and just won't shut up. Hell is here. Hell is in me. I am consumed. Why try again? Why feel hope when time itself has proven that there's no place for me?

Why do I push on just to feel more pain? What am I, crazy?

Better yet, please answer this. Who am I? And what the hell am I doing? In the words of the rapper Tupac Shakur, "I believe hell is coming back to this hopeless life, body and soul reincarnated."

Screw not knowing. I don't want to know anymore. Screw success, for I have no knowledge of what it is. Forget hope, 'cause hope just lets you down. Forget God. He's a wanna-be in a world he knows nothing about. And forget potential. Because without a compass to guide me, what's the point?

We continued talking about his darker times, including the night he walked in a cemetery after midnight and talked to the graves.

"Stop," I said, digging out my digital recorder. "I want to make sure I get this." I laid the recorder on the table and pressed the red record button.

It was all very ghoulish, but then I knew what kind of demons could make somebody want to do such a thing. I waggled my tongue outside my mouth, and twisted my neck until it cracked like dry twigs under a truck tire, and pressure pumped up the front of my head like an air hose.

"You need more time?" Jeff asked.

"What?" I said, hitting pause.

"Are you up for this?"

"Yeah, I'm good," I said, balling my hand into a fist and whacking the front of my forehead twice in a row. "Let's just go on."

Jeff balled his hand into a fist and imitated me, whacking his forehead twice, as I had.

"That's good," he said. "I like that one."

"Oh, you like that?" I said.

"Yeah."

"Well that's my move," I said. "Get your own."

Jeff smiled, then threw a black pen cap at me.

"Hey," I said, putting up a warning finger. "No assaulting the author. I can make you look any way I want."

"Oooh," Jeff said, smiling and throwing up his hands as if to say "I'm soo scared."

We sat at a small table in a room with glass walls in the John Carroll library. I shook my head, then glanced over my shoulder to see if anyone had noticed.

Dork alert! I thought. *Spaz under glass!*

It wasn't as if Jeff cared what I did. There wasn't another person on the planet who understood what was going on with my body better than he did. When it came to tics, he had done everything I had done, and more. But not any longer. And that's why we were sitting there. Jeff was a miracle man—my personal hero—the bravest person I had ever met.

"Ow," I said, grabbing the back of my neck.

"You're sure you want to continue?" he said. "I mean, *you know* I understand."

"Yeah, yeah, you're a freakin' six-foot-five Mother Teresa," I said, stretching. "I'll be fine. Now you can't just leave me in the cemetery. What was it, again? You were talking to dead people?"

In a flash the searing pain in my neck suddenly shot up the back of my skull. I interlaced the fingers of both hands and put them on top of my head and pushed down as hard as I could as if trying to keep it from boring its way through the top my head. I grimaced and closed my eyes. When I opened them I saw Jeff bending forward and staring at me.

"What?" I said, making a circular motion with my hand. "Go! Go!"

"All right," he said. "As long as you promise if it gets too much for you to handle, you'll let me know. Deal?"

I saluted. "Aye, aye, Cap'n."

He threw the pen cap at me again and leaned in closer with an I'm-not-kidding look. "Seriously, Jim."

I shook, then grabbed my long, silver Sony recorder and aimed it at him like a gun. "Talk," I ordered.

He pursed his lips and scooted forward in his chair. "All right, but remember, you asked for it," he said, stretching his arms and arching his back.

It was 11:00 AM. We'd been talking since 7:30. When he stretched, unfolding in every direction like a Swiss Army knife, it struck me how large he really was. He was supersized from his hands and his fingers to his head and torso. Dressed in a blue Nike running suit, he looked strong, tall, and lean with crazy long arms and legs. His bowling-ball-black hair and strong chin framed large brown eyes and a big, goofy Up-with-People smile. Fifteen years my junior, he looked like I used to feel—young, vibrant, and like he could run for an hour without breaking a sweat.

I fought back a yawn as he started to talk. "I'm listening," I said, waving off the yawn. "Just go."

"OK," he said. He looked at me, then looked down. Ten seconds went by before he took a breath and started talking again. "It was 2002," he said. "A very low moment in my life."

As he talked, I found myself in that cemetery with him. "I was driving my green Dodge Spirit that my father had given me. I took that car at night on a fall evening. Fall is my least favorite season because it reminds me of very depressing times. It's gray and everything seems dull. I took a drive to Lakeview Cemetery, which is located right down Mayfield Road in Cleveland, right before you get to Little Italy, about ten minutes from University Hospitals. It's a very old and historic cemetery. Some presidents are buried there. I went alone, without telling anyone I was leaving. I walked through the cemetery, and I walked at a very slow pace. I was wearing a black pair of shiny running pants and a red running coat with black sleeves and a zip-up collar and Adidas high-tops. And as I walked through this cemetery I was talking to the graves."

"To the headstones?" I asked.

"I was talking to the dead," Jeff said. "I was talking to them and trying to find some way to find answers either through myself, within myself, or—hell—if the dead would speak to me, I would have loved to hear it. And as I was talking I would pass by tombs and look at them. I would pay particular attention to the dates of people who died very young. And when I found a date that was around my age, or two or three years older or younger than I was, I was particularly fond of that grave because I didn't want to be in this world anymore. I was jealous that name said Jones or Smith 'cause I wanted it to say Matovic. I wanted it to say 1973–2002, JEFFREY P. MATOVIC. "

He prayed he could switch places with them. It made sense. They could still be enjoying their lives, and he could escape his hell on earth.

"I'd just stand there with my hands in my pockets and stare at the tombstone, and stare at the dates and think about myself being six feet down in a coffin, being cold. But that didn't bother me because that's just a physical body. And I knew if that was me down there below that dirt that I would be in heaven with my grandparents."

"What else do you remember?" I asked.

"I remember kneeling down at a tombstone, and as I knelt with both knees on the soggy, wet ground, I placed my hands in a praying position on the tombstone of this person who I didn't know. The name was Jeffrey P. Orwell, born 1973, died 2001. Close enough, I thought. I knelt down, put my hands on top of the tombstone like I was supporting it [and] giving it love." He interlaced his fingers and demonstrated how he put his palms on the top of the tombstone.

"And then I prayed out loud," he said. "God, why did you take this person and not reserve this spot for me?" he asked.

He rose from the gravestone and stared deeply into the nothingness of the night. Except for the pain of his tics, he was empty inside. A cold wind blew in the echoing silence as he wiped his moist, red eyes and walked back to his car.

24

Luvox, Klonopin, and a Suit to Be Buried In

"POISON CONTROL."

On the day Jeff decided to kill himself, dread coursed through his stomach like a knot of rattlesnakes. Staring at an open pill bottle, he called the Greater Cleveland Poison Control Center and pretended to be a panic-stricken father.

"It's my son!" he said. "I think he's taken thirty Klonopin pills! What do I do? Could that be a lethal dose?"

"Yes sir. That definitely can be very harmful. You should take your son to an emergency room right now. How old is the child?"

"Thank you," Jeff said.

"It might be better to call 9-1-1. How close are you to the nearest ER?"

"Thank you," Jeff said. "I have to go now."

After hanging up the phone, he walked to his closet, then back to his bed. Carefully he laid out his dark blue suit—the suit he wanted to be buried in.

His tics had become too much. *Life* had become too much. He had run into rude people all day who made fun of him. They pointed at him, laughed at him, mocked him behind his back and straight to his face. Worse, his obsessive-compulsive disorder was out of control. He couldn't open his eyes without being obsessed with calculating the midpoints of random objects.

Besides, what was the point of life anyway? To suffer? Because it seemed like that's all he had been doing lately.

It was early 2001 and something terrible had shaken Jeff to his core. His beloved Grandpa Matovic had died the previous September. It hit him like a bolt out of the blue. He had never lost a loved one before. The news did more than leave a hole in his heart. It sent him into a wild, spiraling depression, the likes of which he had never seen.

He always told himself: "If I could just be half the man he is, I will have succeeded greatly in this life." His grandpa was the epitome of the John Carroll motto—he was "a man for others." In many ways his Grandpa Matovic was his hero. He wore well-worn, soft flannel shirts. He was a teddy bear. His hugs were special. He would hold you and he wouldn't let go until you would. Jeff had never hugged anyone and felt that much love passing between them. It was almost like you were getting embraced by the spirit of God and enfolded in his love.

Jeff talked to his grandpa all the time and went to visit him. He had been in assisted living. One day he grabbed a newspaper, got his coffee, and sat down in his favorite recliner. Then he had a heart attack and died—just like that. He was Jeff's first grandparent to die. He was always his favorite grandparent.

And to know that that relationship was gone just annihilated Jeff's hopes and sent him spiraling downward.

Now Jeff *hated* the world. He couldn't stand to look outside and see happy people. It wasn't fair. The world was out to cheat him. God was cruel. He had not only given him Tourette's and OCD, now he had taken his favorite grandfather too? How much was he supposed to be able to take?

Jeff hated all the meaningless clichés that people tossed his way. "Things will get better," they said. "Hang in there."

Hang in there? Jeff thought. *Fucking hang in there?* He was in so much emotional and physical pain he was convinced that it must have been visibly radiating off of him. He felt like saying, "What's wrong with you? Can't you see my pain? Don't you know how much I'm dealing with?"

He said that to his own parents. "Jeff," they'd respond, "we just don't know how to help you. But we'll try to get you someone who can."

"I don't want help!" he screamed. "Nobody can help me! Nobody can fix anything. That's it! Period!"

His mother cried. She'd sit with him in a dark wooden rocking chair in the dining room of their Bay Village home and put her head on his shoulder.

"Whatever help you need," she said. "Just tell me. I'll either give it to you myself, or I will find someone who can give it to you. I just love you so much," she said in a tremulous voice, with tears rolling down her face. "I am trying every minute to understand what you are going through. I would sacrifice my *life* if it would get you the help that you need to ensure your safety, and help you achieve all that you've wanted."

His dad would hold him too, and look at his boy with tears streaming down his face as he firmly gripped his shoulders. "You're the toughest son of a gun that I've ever met!" he said. "I'm so proud of you. Look at what you did at John Carroll!" His voice dropped to a whisper. "You did what people said you'd *never do*. You proved all those assholes wrong!"

Jeff didn't care about the assholes. He didn't care about John Carroll. It was as if he had blinders on. All he cared about was making the pain go away. Desperate to end his suffering, he picked up his plastic prescription bottle and poured a pile of multicolored meds into his palm—both Luvox and Klonopin. One by one they were a prison; all at once they were freedom. It was a powerful thought. Liberating.

Try and stop this, Tourette's! "Stupid life!" he cried out loud. Jeff gulped the pills, as many and as fast as he could, cramming them down his throat as if plunging a silver dagger into the heart of his pain.

Immediately afterward, though, Jeff stood up and snatched the phone in a panic. He was so confused. He didn't *really* want to die. It just felt so good to finally take some action, to strike out, to do *something* rather than just take it day after day. Groggy, he called his mother as the darkness began to close in around him.

Patty Matovic rushed to her son's apartment. Tasting fear in her mouth, she searched the place, finally finding him, half in bed and half on the floor. She saw the bottle of pills on the nightstand.

"Jeff!" She didn't know if he was alive or dead. With tears in her eyes she shook her son, desperately trying to get some response. He didn't move.

With shaking hands, she picked up the phone and dialed 9-1-1. Minutes later paramedics arrived and took him to the hospital.

25

"Get in Here and Take Care of Me!"

"HEY, YOU FUCKING son of bitch! Get in here and take care of me!" Jeff didn't usually talk like that. He was delusional. Even after getting his stomach pumped at the Cleveland Clinic, the drugs continued to rage through his bloodstream. They caused confusion and paranoia.

"We've got to get your respirations up," he heard a trauma doctor say. "Because if we don't, we could be looking at a very serious problem."

Who was this? And what was going on? For a while he didn't know who he was—or where he was. But one thing was sure. If he hadn't gotten there, he would have died.

Angry, combative, and suspicious, he took his confusion out on his nurses. He called them names, tried to hit them, and screamed when teams of them held him down to give him shots or force the liquid charcoal down his throat that burned like battery acid. In his altered state he thought he was under attack.

"What are you giving me?" he screamed.

The nurses tried to calm him, tell him they were there to help. Their words were meaningless. He didn't want to be touched. He felt like a fighter, only he couldn't tell whether he was still slugging it out or if he had already been knocked out.

He spent three days in the hospital—the three worst days of his life. As his body began to process the chemical soup in his system, his severe withdrawal symptoms scared him more than anything he had ever faced. Frigidly cold, colder than he had ever been in his life, his body shook so hard he rattled the side of his bed. Even after nurses covered him with six hospital blankets, he continued to shiver. It felt like he was lying naked in the snow. The only thing that made sense in his confusion and discomfort was to yell as loudly as he could for help.

"I just want to talk to my dad!" he screamed. "Get my dad on the phone—*now*! Call him at work and tell him his son needs to talk to him."

It was 3:00 AM. Time had no meaning in the haze of his drug-addled brain. After his body stabilized and the drugs left his system, he was released.

He felt lucky to be alive. After all, he really didn't want to die.

It was one of the biggest mistakes of his life. In the months that followed he realized how foolish he had been and how much it would have hurt his family if he had died. Slowly he refocused himself and regained the will to live.

26

"Nice Boots!"

IN HIS LATE twenties, Jeff got a job working with severely autistic kids at the Cleveland Clinic Foundation's Children's Center for Rehabilitation. His job gave him both a steady income and great satisfaction. The kids inspired him, and they didn't care if he ticked.

After months of work he had finally made a breakthrough with a five-year-old nonverbal boy by using behavior modification to get the child to point to pictures in sequence to communicate the phrase, "I like to play at recess."

Jeff smiled broadly as he sat across a desk from the blond-haired, blue-eyed boy. "Recess?" he said, using the picture book to give his response. "Me too!" He pointed to pictures in sequence to say, "Let's play ball at recess."

The rail-thin boy smiled in return. It was essentially his first successful communication. Jeff had taken a special interest in the boy and worked hard with him. He even researched special techniques on his own time.

Jeff stayed with his uncle Paul and aunt Karen in the Cleveland suburb of South Euclid while he looked for an apartment nearer to his job. Life was far from perfect, but it was as good as it could be considering his serious tics. Medications helped—most of the time. His job at the center kept him busy and distracted. That helped hold his tics in check. Sure, he had his dark days. But other days were good. August 20, 2002, was *great*.

Done for the day, he waved good-bye to his coworkers. Dressed in khakis, leather dress shoes, and a blue, three-button, short-sleeved polo with the rehab center's logo on the left breast, he felt good as he walked to the Rapid, Cleveland's light-rail train. Jeff didn't have a car. The reasons were more than financial. While he could drive, he didn't trust himself to do it all the time. Every day after work he took the green line to his stop in Eastern Cleveland, just outside of Shaker Heights, where he caught a bus home. He made the same trip every day.

But on Tuesday, August 20, 2002, his commute was anything but ordinary.

— —

DEBRA JANNING WASN'T looking for a man.

The five-foot-three, attractive thirty-three-year-old with the reddish-brown hair had two children—preteens from her first marriage, which ended in divorce in 1995. She had just gotten out of a relationship six months earlier, and she had recently turned down several men who had asked her on dates.

You know something? she thought. *I'm done with men. That's it. I'm going to focus on myself, and my work, and raising my kids.*

She worked as an administrative assistant to the director of sales at the Convention and Visitor's Bureau of Greater Cleveland. She and her kids, eleven-year-old Bonnie and nine-year-old Mike, lived in a duplex on Green Road in South Euclid, right on the bus line. With no money for a car, she took the bus to her stop in Eastern Cleveland, just outside of Shaker Heights.

At the end of the day on August 20, 2002, Debra Janning walked to that same bus stop to go back home. Her kids were spending the week with her ex-husband, who had moved to Toledo after the divorce. Bonnie and Mike would be coming home that weekend.

It was sunny, with just a pinch of autumn in the air, when Debra arrived at the bus stop just after 5:00 PM. She felt good in a new outfit—a crisp black suit with a three-button blazer and a burgundy shirt and mid-cut, black leather zip-up boots not even twenty-four-hours old.

A slight breeze blew as the train doors opened and passengers began stepping off of the green line. Debra's eyes glazed over them all . . . until—

Wait a minute! Her eyes settled on Jeff. He was six-foot-five and athletically slender, with coal-black hair and large white teeth. She had always liked tall men. And this one was *cute*!

At the same time Jeff had taken notice of the petite woman in the sexy black boots sitting on the bus bench with her legs crossed and her hand over her purse. *Wow!* he thought.

She was so pretty and well dressed. She looked like a professional. Better yet, she was alone! Jeff smiled as he walked toward the bench and sat down next to her.

At the time, the cocktail of meds Jeff was on were working well enough so that—over short bursts of time—you wouldn't notice anything was wrong.

To Debra he just seemed charming.

"Nice boots!" he said.

Debra looked down, then smiled shyly. "Who are you, and why do you like my boots?" she said.

"I just like 'em," he said.

They exchanged names. Jeff made her laugh. The small talk was nothing special—but the sparks they felt when they looked into each other's eyes were. He asked about her job, then she about his. They realized neither of them owned a car.

The Number 34 Green Road bus came in four minutes. It seemed like seconds.

Debra stood up when her bus arrived.

"Oh, that's my bus too," Jeff said.

Great, Debra thought. *What a wonderful chance to keep talking to this guy.*

They boarded together. Debra sat down first on one of the bench seats on the right side facing the middle of the bus. There was another seat in front of her and behind her. But to her surprise, Jeff sat down right next to her. They sat together facing a young man in his early twenties on the bench seat on the left side.

The conversation continued, and for fifteen minutes it was as if they were alone on the bus. They couldn't take their eyes off each other. Debra's heart beat faster. There was just something about this guy—his eyes, his smile, his charm.

Debra Janning wasn't looking for a man. But she may have found one. As the bus neared her stop, she handed Jeff her business card with her phone number on the back. "Give me a call sometime," she said.

Jeff took the card and watched her walk off the bus. After she did, the guy in the seat facing him raised his eyebrows and gave Jeff a thumbs-up.

"Smooth move, man!" he said.

— —

BACK HOME, JEFF pulled the card out of his khakis and put it in his wallet. He couldn't stop thinking about the pretty woman in the sexy boots. He called her the next night for a date that weekend. Deb couldn't make it then but they made a date for the next week. In the meantime they continued to see each other at the stop and on the Green Road bus. Jeff was smitten by Debra, a woman as smart and interesting as she was sassy and sexy. They continued talking, and laughing. And the more Debra looked into Jeff's deep brown eyes, the more she felt like she was falling into them, getting lost in them. It was almost like she could see into his soul.

After four days they had their first romantic moment, a tender kiss while sitting in the steel-and-glass bus shelter. It was the most natural kiss Debra had ever experienced. And the electricity was off the scale. If there were people sitting around them, she neither noticed nor cared.

On the night of their first date, Jeff came over to Debra's house, where they watched *Beauty and the Beast* with her kids and ordered a hand-tossed cheese pizza from Marco's. It wasn't anything fancy, but for Jeff and Debra it felt right. They had fun just being around each other, and neither felt pressure to be someone they weren't.

Debra lived on the second floor of a stylish but humid three-bedroom duplex on Green Road. The house had beige walls, seven-foot ceilings, and low-hanging ceiling fans. Many times the former basketball player would forget the fans were there and take a spinning blade to the forehead. After the kids went to bed, Debra and Jeff walked down to the first floor and out to her landlady's front porch. Debra usually didn't go there. But it was such a nice evening that she made an exception. She sat with Jeff on the porch swing with blue-and-white striped cushions.

For their second date, Jeff borrowed his uncle's car, an older four-door sedan. He took Debra to the Improv, a comedy club on the West Bank of Cleveland's Flats. He showed up at Debra's door in a suit carrying a bouquet of summer flowers. She answered the door in a little black dress.

While Debra enjoyed Jeff's company, it wasn't long before she noticed his curious collection of shakes, blinks, twitches, and sounds. While she wondered about them, they weren't bad enough to scare her off. She had seen tics before. In high school she had worked in her father's medical office and had seen many nice people with many odd problems. She herself had worn braces on her legs when she was a toddler. Her father, a podiatrist, taught her never to judge people by their medical issues, but to look inside. The more Debra looked at who Jeff was inside, the more she fell for him. They began spending a lot of time together. The more comfortable he became, the more his fun and playful personality came out. Not long into their relationship, Debra's kids had grown close to Jeff too.

Since both Jeff and Debra were strapped for cash and neither had a car, they spent a lot of time at home or walking to nearby parks with the kids. Over Labor Day weekend Debra invited Jeff to a family barbecue at her cousin Betty's house. Thanks to his medication, Jeff managed to keep his tics in check long enough to make a good impression. One of Debra's cousins brought a horse to the gathering. The children soon glommed onto the tall new stranger, taking turns asking him to put them on the horse. Debra watched the gentle and charming way Jeff played with the kids and interacted with her cousin Nancy.

"Deb," Nancy said. "You've got a good one there. Don't let him get away."

"Don't worry," Debra said. She had fallen in love with him. At the same time, however, Jeff was falling victim to rapidly worsening tics. Deb didn't see them at first. But within weeks after they started dating little things became more apparent—the constant clearing of his throat, spreading his fingers wide apart, facial grimaces, and the explosive arm and leg movements. Debra knew something was wrong. But Jeff was so handsome, and they had so much chemistry, that it didn't matter to her.

It mattered to Jeff. He worried that she would reject him as many others had. Still, he *had* to tell her. He had to be free to tic in front of her, and for her to accept what she was seeing. It was only fair. But how could he tell her? And what would she think of him?

More than a month later, he finally worked up the courage. As they sat together on a white love seat watching a movie, he paused it and took her hand. He put his right leg on the cushion and turned his body to face her. Then he put his left hand gently on top of her right.

"We have to talk," he said.

Uh-oh. Debra thought he was breaking up with her.

Jeff locked his eyes on hers. "There's something I really need to tell you," he said, as his right leg began to twitch. "I was born with a condition that causes motor and vocal tics. Do you know what a tic is?"

"Yes," she said. "Some of my dad's patients had movement disorders that caused tics."

"Well," Jeff said. "The condition I have is called Tourette Syndrome." Jeff cocked his head and smiled. "It can't kill me. But it does cause me to have arm or leg tics that can be very noticeable, especially in stressful situations. And sometimes the heat can cause them to flare up, or even changes in the weather."

He leaned in. "Do you know what Tourette Syndrome is? Because I want to want to make sure you don't stereotype it like the public does as the 'swearing disease.'"

"Yes," she said. "I'm aware of what Tourette's is, and I know how the public misperceives it. But tell me more about it."

Jeff sighed. She hadn't freaked out. She hadn't thrown him down the stairs. *And she wanted to know more!*

He put on his teacher's hat. "Tourette's is a neurological chemical imbalance in the brain in a location called the basal ganglia . . ." he started.

Debra relaxed her body and put her arm on the back of the sofa as she engaged more fully in the conversation. After fifteen minutes of talking, Debra said, "Yeah. I've noticed sometimes you'll extend your fingers out and stretch them. It looks painful. I've also noticed that sometimes you blink your eyes quickly. I always assumed your eyes were just dry."

"Good," Jeff said. "I'm glad that you've seen them. I've wanted to tell you for so long, but I was scared and I didn't want to be rejected—again. Especially after I've fallen so deeply in love with you."

"They don't matter to me," Debra said, reaching out to enfold his hand in hers. "And I love you too. I love you for who you are *inside*."

Jeff closed his eyes and took a big breath. It was as if someone had just lifted a thousand-pound weight off his shoulders and erased a lifetime of bad memories.

"Really?" he said, smiling at her. They fell into each other's arms in a soft embrace.

JEFF AND DEBRA dated for another month before Jeff moved out of his uncle Paul's apartment and into his own place in Shaker Heights in September 2002. It was exciting. For the first time in a long time, things were looking up. He had a job, money in the bank, and he'd fallen in love with a beautiful woman. And now he was getting his own apartment!

For the first time in his life he felt truly free. This was *his* time, he thought. The sun was out, the sky was blue, and nothing could hold him back—not even his Tourette's. With a positive outlook for the days ahead, he paid the landlord in cash and moved in.

He wished that the positive feeling he had about his life would last forever.

It didn't.

A month later, the dark clouds that had parted so quickly for him began to roll back in just as fast.

27

"Jeff, It's Deb. Where Are You?"

DEPRESSION COVERED JEFF like a blanket. He knew Debra had developed feelings for him, and he for her. He dropped his head. It wouldn't last. It *couldn't*.

You're going to mess it up, he told himself. *You're going to be a failure, just like always!*

She didn't know the *real* him. The voices in his head grew louder and more insistent. *You're a fraud, Jeff. A fraud!*

He wasn't worthy of her love. And what right did he have to drag her into his secret world of pain? Sure, she knew he had tics. But she didn't know how ugly they could get. She didn't know *anything*!

As his desperation grew more dangerous, Jeff did little to make his new place a home. He didn't *deserve* a nice place. He didn't furnish it or clean it. Before long the one-room apartment became dingy. Normally a very clean person, Jeff stopped bathing and washing his clothes. His apartment had become a prison. The heat and electricity didn't work, and he didn't even care if the landlord ever fixed them.

Let's face it, he thought, *I'm a nobody. A born loser.* The best he could do was survive one more day in the dark and the cold.

He dropped out of sight, didn't go to Debra's house anymore, didn't return her phone calls. And he wouldn't answer his door. He wouldn't even call his own mom and dad, even after they left numerous messages pleading for him to do so. He felt infected, and he didn't want to spread his sickness—even over the phone.

Debra was confused, worried. She left numerous e-mails and phone messages. "Jeff, are you all right?" she said. "Jeff, it's Deb. Where are you? Why won't you call me back?" Weeks passed.

When Jeff finally called Debra back, he was not himself. He seemed distant, odd. "I'm not going to be able to see you anymore," he said. "I'm joining the navy."

Jeff was not eating, exercising, or leaving his dirty apartment by this time. He had cut off all social interaction. Not only was he not in his right state of mind, he began believing things that weren't true.

"The *navy?*" Debra said, perplexed.

"Yeah," Jeff said. "I applied several months ago. They're putting me into a secret program. My phones are going to be tapped, and I'm not going to be able to see or talk to anybody for quite some time."

"What?" Debra said. It didn't make any sense. Jeff never said anything about going into the navy. With his bad knee and the severity of his tics, the navy would *never* let him join. Besides—had he forgotten? They had planned a life together. Debra's mind raced. What was wrong? What had happened to him?

The next day Debra had a friend watch her kids and took a taxi to Jeff's apartment. Worried, she knocked on the door.

No answer.

She stepped back and saw movement through a window. Frantic, she banged on the door. "Jeff! Come down here and talk to me," she yelled. "Tell me what's going on."

He never did.

It was likely a problem with his medications, she thought. An overdose, an underdose, or perhaps a drug interaction. Concerned, she called Jeff's parents.

"Mrs. Matovic," she said that evening, "my name is Debra Janning, and I've been dating your son."

Debra could almost hear the "Oh no" in the silence on the other end. Then Patty said, "Hold on a second. Jim! Get on the phone."

Debra swallowed hard. "First off I want to tell you what an incredibly wonderful, caring, loving son you have," she said. "I think he's the most wonderful man in the world. But there's something going on here that I'm concerned about." Debra recounted the strange events.

Patty Matovic said she'd call her brother, Paul, who lived in South Euclid to go check on Jeff. The next day Paul knocked on Jeff's door and got lucky. Jeff knew it wasn't Debra or his parents, so he thought it might be safe. Besides, he hadn't collected his mail for several weeks.

Once inside, Paul knew right away something was very wrong. Jeff was naturally clean and tidy, to the point of obsessiveness. But his apartment was filthy. Even more worrisome, Jeff himself appeared incoherent and had not shaved or bathed in several days.

Paul called Jeff's parents, who came immediately and drove him to the emergency room. He was sent to Laurelwood, a mental health satellite branch of University Hospitals, for a seventy-two-hour psychiatric observation.

When Jim Matovic visited his son at Laurelwood, his heart sank. It was frightening to see his youngest child in a padded room with everything stripped away that he possibly could use to cause himself harm. There were no strings or cords of any kind. They had even removed the cloth tie around his bathrobe.

Jeff's father tried to smile, but all he could think was how heartwrenching it was. He kept the visit short. What could he say other than he loved him?

After three days Jeff was released, but he was not allowed to go back to his apartment. He stayed with family for more than half a year. At his doctor's urging he enrolled in an intensive class to learn something called dialectical behavioral therapy. The class, the doctor told him, would help him better deal with tics and the stress of his increasingly difficult life. Jeff took the doctor's advice. The class helped him to think more clearly and not act so impulsively. It gave him an emotional tool belt to deal with stressful situations so that they wouldn't spiral out of control.

A week before Christmas 2002, Jeff called Deb and said he wanted to celebrate graduating from his dialectical behavioral therapy class. And he told her he had found a little calico cat and named her Leah. Knowing how much Deb loved cats, Jeff asked her for advice on properly caring for his new pet. Debra could hear it in his voice. Her Jeff was back.

Not long afterward, Deb let Jeff stay at her place. A day turned into two, which turned into a week. Eventually they decided to make it permanent.

In January 2003, Jeff moved in with Debra for good.

28

"How Much Do You Love Me?"

LIVING WITH DEBRA proved to be just what Jeff needed. They watched movies together, played basketball, went out for pizza, and stayed home laughing and talking. As the months passed, their relationship deepened. They had fallen deeply in love.

On the night of April 3, 2003, Jeff told Debra he was taking her out for ice cream. Except he wasn't. It was just a ruse to get her out of the house. Instead of stopping at an ice cream parlor, the couple stopped at a Catholic church known as St. Greg's to say a prayer for Jeff's knee surgery the next day. Alone in the sanctuary in the early evening, they prayed as the sun streamed playfully through the stained-glass windows in the eighty-one-year-old gothic church.

Sitting in a pew near the front, the couple started talking quietly about their lives, reminiscing about times that had brought them closer. Jeff rested his folded hands on the pew in front of him. He stared at the church's crucifix in silence for several minutes. Debra placed her hand on his right knee.

"Whenever you're done, just let me know," she whispered. "But certainly there's no rush." When they got up from the pews and headed toward the exit, Jeff reached out to grab Debra's left hand as they passed a table full of prayer candles.

"Hold on a second," he said in a serious but calm voice.

Debra turned until she was facing him.

"You know that I love you so very much, and have cherished every moment I have spent with you," he said.

"I feel the same way," she said.

"Debra?" Jeff said, pausing for effect. "How much do you love me?"

He knew the answer. "Fifty cents!" she said with a smile.

It was the same answer he used to give to his mother as a young boy when he thought fifty cents was just about the largest fortune he could imagine.

Debra took his hands and repeated her answer. "Fifty cents!" she said. "A *million* dollars!"

"Well, here's how much I love you," Jeff said, getting down on his one knee and pulling a sparkling diamond engagement ring out of his pocket. "*This* much."

She covered her mouth with her hands.

"Yes!" she said through her tears, throwing her arms around him. "Oh *yes*!"

THE WORD OF the engagement spread quickly. Jeff and Debra were planning a life together.

By this time Jeff had met Debra's parents and spent time with them. Recently they had all gone to dinner with Deb's aunt Jean at the Brown Derby, a steak restaurant in Cleveland where the local custom was cracking fresh, ballpark peanuts at your table, then tossing the shells on the floor.

Mike Janning, Debra's father, was a good judge of character. Jeff was clearly a good man who loved his little girl. But when he saw Jeff's tics, he couldn't help but wonder—as a father and a physician—if love would be enough. While he and Debra ran an errand together, he turned to her in his car.

"Debra," he said in his best concerned father voice. "Are you . . . sure about Jeff?" He talked about his tics and how difficult life could become if they got worse. He talked in stark terms. These things can be hell to live with, he told her. And they can change and make your life harder than you could possibly imagine.

And so he asked her again. "Are you sure?"

Debra put her hand on his shoulder. "I'm sure, Dad," she said.

"But his tics . . ."

"I'm *sure*, Dad. I don't care about his tics."

"Do you love him?"

"Very much," she said.

Mike Janning sighed and gazed far out the window, still not sure himself. "Well," he finally said, "as long as you've thought about this."

29

A Little Beige on the Side

JEFF AND DEBRA eagerly started planning their future together. They talked about getting married at the Great Lakes Renaissance Fair in the summer of 2004 in Rock Creek, about an hour outside of Cleveland. And in early August 2003, they moved from Debra's small apartment on Green Road to a two-story rental house in Lyndhurst.

The large white house felt like a palace by comparison. It had a full living room, a full dining room, and a large great room. There were three bedrooms upstairs and a finished rec room and workshop downstairs. Built in the 1950s, it had dark hardwood floors, a hoop in the driveway, and a wooden fence around the backyard. Morning and afternoon sun poured through new windows in the great room, while the living room sported a light brown window seat under a bay window. Virtually everything was new in the large kitchen, and the gorgeous light brown oak cabinets made Debra smile.

Little by little they began to make the house their own. One Saturday they decided to paint their bedroom beige. Jeff wore an old John Carroll T-shirt, a pair of paint-spattered navy gym shorts, and old white tennis shoes stained green from mowing the lawn. Deb wore old blue jeans and a white paint shirt. They laid down a clear sheet of plastic to protect the hardwood floor and began to paint the walls. Debra smiled as she painted.

"What?" Jeff said, looking back at her.

"It's just going to feel so good to get everything the way *we* want it. I can't wait until we get this done. We already have the paint for Bonnie's bedroom and your office. Do you still want the accent wall in your office to be hunter green?"

"That'd be great," Jeff said. "We can go pick that up tomorrow morning."

As they continued painting, Jeff quipped, "You know that green wall may just give us luck and make us rich," he said. "It *is* the color of money!"

"Yeah, right!" Deb said. "When Ed McMahon shows up on our doorstep on Saturday morning, *then* I'll believe it."

"Hey, a guy can dream for miracles, can't he?"

Deb smiled and shook her head. "Sure," she said. "Why not?"

By the middle of the afternoon they had both made good progress on their walls. But with all his hard work, Jeff soon overheated. That sent his tics into warp drive. His right leg began thumping against the wooden floor so hard it rattled the lights in the living room. He let out a series of five explosive grunts. His eyes opened wide, before blinking shut hard. His nose scrunched like a bunny's and his mouth grimaced and contorted.

"You want to stop now, babe?" Deb said. "Get a drink of water?"

"Nah, I'm all right. Just let me just take a breath. I'll be fine."

"OK. But after we finish let's go down and grab a sandwich and have a nice lunch."

"Yeah . . . sounds good."

But painting a wall when his Tourette's was acting up was difficult at best. Jeff loaded his roller with beige paint and pressed it to the wall with his right hand. But before he could start rolling, a savage tic caused that arm to jerk backward with a violent twitch. With all the force he could muster, he flung a large blob of beige paint over his left shoulder, tagging Debra square in the back between her shoulder blades with a loud splat!

Oh God! Jeff turned around quickly to see where the paint had gone. Did he hit the ceiling? Had he tossed some out in the hallway?

Nope.

Slowly, Debra reached over her right shoulder and felt the splotch of paint. With her mouth and eyes wide open in surprise, she turned around and extended her hands as if to say, "Oh you *did not* just do that!" Then Debra showed Jeff a side of her he had never seen—an exciting, childlike side that he liked very much. Wearing a wicked smile, she glared at the brush she had just loaded with beige paint and said, "Oh yeah? Well, take *this*!"

She flipped the brush toward Jeff, covering him from chin to shin in fresh beige paint. Jeff looked down at himself and started to laugh. Then he hoisted his roller skyward like a samurai warrior and advanced toward his wide-eyed fiancée. Debra began to squeal as the paint began to fly.

⌒ ⌒

FOR A WHILE, living together was wonderful. For the most part, the medications were keeping the tics in check. Jeff and Debra were genuinely happy. Only one thing could threaten their future together: Jeff's tics, which over the long, hot summer battered him like a hurricane. Jeff hung on valiantly, but it wasn't enough. Before long he began losing the battle.

Debra knew she loved Jeff and wanted to marry him. But over the next few months, life with him became so hard that she began to wonder whether she could.

30

Debra's Dilemma

JEFF'S TICS CONTINUED to worsen. They were more frequent now and had more than doubled in strength from just a few months ago. To make matters worse, new tics had emerged. Years ago he'd have just gone to the doctor for different pills, new combinations of pills, or an adjustment to the dosage of his old pills. And to be fair that *had* helped—at least for a while. But after nearly twenty years, after ingesting a pharmacy full of medications, he grew tired of the game, sick of well-meaning, pill-pushing doctors who offered him kind words and warmed-over platitudes wrapped in a yet another prescription label instead of any real hope.

Pills? Yeah, he had done pills. Blue pills, white pills, red pills, capsules, caplets, soft-gels, time-release tabs. Most weren't even designed for people with Tourette's. They were tranquilizers, old blood pressure medications, and antipsychotic drugs adapted to some new, never-designed-for role. But what could he do? That's what the doctors recommended. So day after day that's what he did: throw down the dope. Swallow and hope.

Truth is, even when the pills worked, they didn't work that well. And now they weren't working at all. Alone against the growing evil inside of him, he tried every way imaginable to stay still—relaxation, deep-breathing exercises, meditation, prayer, primal screams . . .

It didn't matter. The evil was winning. It assumed control over every part of his body like some sort of satanic puppet master. If it was just one that was twitching—his head, or his arm—he could adjust or take measures to control it. But these tics were too frequent and too strong. Refusing to be contained, they swept across his body like a brush fire, affecting his arms, legs, wrists, ankles, torso, head, neck, eyes, and even his voice. They made him grunt and grimace. They were there in the way he stood and the way he sat. They affected they way he talked, the way he breathed. They even followed him into bed at night, blanketing him with sharp spasms that contorted his body into painful positions, making it next to impossible to quiet his mind enough to fall asleep.

Why was this happening to him? And why didn't it ever seem to happen to anybody else? Lord knows there were all sorts of jerks who deserved to suffer like this. Not him. And certainly not Debra or the kids.

The more he thought about it, the more troubling it became. He wanted so badly to be the man Debra deserved. He wanted to take her out to eat, to go dancing, have a good time. He wanted to laugh and run, to shoot hoops with Bonnie and Mike, to watch movies and play games like he'd been able to just months ago.

The evil wouldn't hear of it. It attacked him like an invisible army, leaving him exhausted, angry, and despondent. Bedridden and largely helpless against its onslaught, he depended more and more on Debra, who had gone from gracious girlfriend to nightly nursemaid.

How did it get this way? Deb wondered. *This bad?* Their home had become a prison of work and self-sacrifice to the all-powerful Tourettan gods. Working full time in the sales department of the hypercompetitive Sheraton Cleveland City Center Hotel was hard enough. But it was nothing compared to the work that remained after Debra got home.

Jeff was little more than an invalid. Debra tried to remember the good times, the times he made her laugh when no one else could, the times he did things that were so sweet it made her cry, the times in the still of the night they told each other things that no one else knew.

She remembered the love in his eyes when he had proposed, the way he complimented her, the way he loved Bonnie and Mike as his own, and that big, broad, wonderful smile.

God he was handsome. And smart. And kind. And funny. But like Debra, he was falling apart. He couldn't dress himself, couldn't eat by himself, couldn't always walk himself to the bathroom, or up to bed, without help.

If that was all there was to taking care of him, maybe she could handle it. But there was so much more. She couldn't watch the news in the morning—or the evening—because it would fire up Jeff's tics. She couldn't talk to him about their financial situation because it would fire up his tics. They couldn't go to movies anymore because it would fire up his tics. Dinner had to be on the table every night at the same time, or it would fire up his tics. And the house had to be spotless—scrubbed, straightened, and orderly—or his obsessive-compulsive disorder would explode, which would in turn fire up his tics.

And finally, the house had to be quiet. No extraneous noise. *Nothing*!

Jeff couldn't stand it. Deb survived second by second. The only thing she could allow herself to think about was what was happening at work or with the kids. She couldn't concern herself too much with what was happening to Jeff or she would have a nervous breakdown.

It was the worst time in their relationship.

One night was harder than all the others. Late in the evening, after Bonnie and Mike had gone to bed, it was Jeff's turn. Debra massaged his back, his neck, his arms and legs, sponging away the sweat and dabbing him with ice bags to cool him down in the summer heat. With enough time and attention, he would finally quiet down enough to sleep out of sheer exhaustion, his body physically unable to sustain the tics that still raged inside.

Well after midnight, Debra finally got something she wanted: an hour or so for herself. She walked downstairs, sunk into the couch, and stared blankly into the inky blackness. And then, slowly, silently, she began to cry.

She loved Jeff and wanted a life with him. And she could never leave him, especially in a time of need. But increasingly she wondered whether she could live with the pressure his worsening tics continued to place on her.

She couldn't go forward. She couldn't go back. And she couldn't keep going like she was. As days blurred into nights, and nights into days, the workload rarely ceased. Debra had always been strong. But now even her resolve was fading. With no other option, she turned to God.

"Why is this happening?" she demanded, begging for help one moment, yelling the next. Deep inside, she feared the situation would never change. This would be her life with Jeff. This, or worse. For fifty years.

"Oh, God!" The world began closing in on her.

There, in the darkness, in the desperation and the pain, a horrible but fleeting thought flashed through her mind. *Maybe,* she thought, *it would be better if I just went upstairs and killed him.*

"NO!" she said immediately, brushing it from her mind like a bad dream. What was she thinking? She could never do that, no matter how bad he got. She loved him too much.

But then what could she do?

Crying, she burrowed deeper into the couch and pulled her grandfather's robe tight. "Grandma and Grandpa," she said in a small voice, "you've got to help me. You've got to show me that everything is going to be OK."

Just then she began to smell the sweet smoke of her grandfather's pipe tobacco and feel the hands of her grandmother softly stroking her hair.

Her grandparents had passed away years ago.

31

Learn to Live with Your Pain

"HEY! YOU'RE NOT allowed back there!" The secretary glared at the interloper. Jeff didn't care. He was on a mission, and nobody was going to stop him. Walking fast, he blew past the woman into the empty office of one of the Cleveland Clinic's most prominent neurosurgeons.

"You can't just barge in there like that!" she said.

"Nah, that's good," Jeff said. "I'm fine." He placed a letter in the center of the surgeon's desk. Then he took a yellow Post-it Note and wrote "Urgent! Read Now!!!" in red pen, and stuck it on top of the letter. Not that it would do any good. He just didn't know what else to do.

For thirty years Jeff had been respectful and played by the rules. That had gotten him nowhere. Day after day he'd been told that a neurosurgeon would call him back. They never did.

The time for rule following was over. This time it was "Get out of my way, I'm coming through!"

The severity of Jeff's tics had been varying wildly over the last few months. Sometimes he could walk and talk, other days he was bedridden and functionally mute. Desperate to find an answer, he had researched possible solutions and settled on deep brain stimulation as the most promising option. He asked his neurologist about it, but there was a problem. As he aged he had to move from Dr. Erenberg—a pediatric neurologist whom he loved—to an adult neurologist whom he didn't. His new doctor consistently refused to give him a referral to see a neurosurgeon. He only suggested more pills, or different pills—which was a problem.

The pills weren't working anymore.

Finally, in August 2003, he scheduled a special meeting with his neurologist. The doctor, in his mid-sixties with salt-and-pepper hair, sat at his desk quietly taking notes. "So how are we doing today?" he said, using his stock phrase.

The man never leaned forward. He would always lean backward and tilt his notes toward himself. The way Jeff saw it, he dismissed Jeff's concerns as easily as you'd brush a fly off your shoulders. He was smart, Jeff felt, but empathetically bankrupt.

In a calm but determined voice, as his tics caused him to jerk and flail, Jeff asked for—then insisted on—a referral to see a neurosurgeon.

"Jeff," his exasperated doctor said, looking up from his chart. "I won't write you a referral simply because," he paused for emphasis, "you wouldn't be a person they'd accept."

Jeff knew why. It was his suicide attempt. One stupid decision and now doctors had made up their mind about him. He had been medically stereotyped. It was as if he had been wrapped with yellow police tape that read: CAUTION. PSYCH PATIENT. APPROACH AT YOUR OWN RISK.

He felt labeled, trapped. He wasn't crazy, just in *pain*. Couldn't they understand that? But the more desperate he became, the crazier he looked. Turned down for the referral yet again, the conversation grew heated.

Finally, his doctor had had enough. "You know what, Jeff," he said. "I don't know what else to do for you. We've tried the therapies, we've tried the medicines, and we've tried different combinations of medicines and therapies." He did everything but throw up his hands.

Jeff didn't know what to think. He was giving up on him? Was that it? He felt a deep emptiness inside.

"So you're telling me, Doctor, that you're out of ideas for me?" he said. "That I'm out of options?" He stared at the suddenly impotent healer with shocked sadness. "So what am I supposed to do now?" he asked.

His doctor pursed his lips for several seconds. "I'm sorry," he said. "You'll just . . . have to learn to live with your pain."

Jeff pulled back.

Live with his pain? That's the one thing he couldn't do. *Wouldn't* do!

Jeff got up as the doctor closed his chart. "Thanks for your time, Doc," he said curtly, barely bothering to hide his anger. Ticked, he rode the elevator to the lobby. Stopping at a pay phone, he looked up the number for the Cleveland Clinic's archrival—University Hospitals—and called it. Located less than five miles from each other, the two hospitals competed with each other for grant money and reputation.

A receptionist put him through to a woman named Arlene Brown, secretary for Dr. Robert Maciunas. "Department of Neurosurgery, may I help you?" she said in a caring voice.

"Hi, my name is Jeff Matovic," Jeff said. "Look, Arlene. I am having a *really* hard time with my Tourette Syndrome. I know you know what that is."

"Yes," she said. "I'm very familiar with Tourette's."

"Well, I am in dire straits. I am currently at the Cleveland Clinic. I've been a patient here since the early '80s, and I have needs that can't be met here. They are unwilling to cooperate on any basis. I am possibly seeking some help looking for a surgery technique. Does your surgeon perform deep brain stimulation?"

"Yes," Brown said.

"When can I see him?"

Jeff wasn't expecting much. His mind imagined a worst-case scenario. *Uhh, we're pretty booked up for the next five years, so . . .*

The real response was better than he could have dreamed. "Does two weeks from now on Monday sound good to you?"

Jeff's eyes grew large. He started breathing faster as he shifted in his seat. Had he heard right?

"Two weeks?" he said.

"Yes sir."

"You bet!" he said, circling the date in red in his planner. "I'll be there! Thank you!"

He let the name roll around in his mind. "Ma-*soon*-us" he said, repeating Arlene Brown's pronunciation. "Dr. Robert Ma-*soon*-us."

He turned around and took one final look at the lobby of the Cleveland Clinic. He had been a patient there for twenty years. But now it was over. In his mind he was wiping the slate clean, starting over. He couldn't believe it. *Finally* he was going to see a neurosurgeon! *Finally* he was going to ask for deep brain stimulation! *Finally* his years of research just might pay off.

There was just one problem: Dr. Maciunas could still say no.

32

Take a Chance on Me

HOURS SEEMED LIKE days. As he stared at his black leather planner with the date of his meeting circled in red, Jeff wished he could take a sleeping pill and wake up two weeks later in Dr. Maciunas's office.

He calculated the time remaining. Two weeks. Fourteen days. Three hundred thirty-six hours. Twenty thousand one hundred and sixty minutes.

Do I have twenty thousand minutes to my death? he wondered. He swallowed hard.

Even as Jeff prepared a presentation to persuade Dr. Maciunas to say yes, he researched ways to kill himself in case the doctor said no. He couldn't take another rejection. This was it. Last chance.

Jeff didn't know what Maciunas would say. But he did know he couldn't keep living like this. Tourette's possessed his body like an evil spirit, forcing his arms to stick out, zombielike. The vicious ticking pulled muscles and tendons, cracked joints and bones. The disorder completely engulfed him. He had lost himself. Subsumed into the tics, he ceased being Jeff Matovic and had *become* his Tourette's.

Everything hurt. He hadn't had a good night's sleep in more than a month. And no matter what he did, he couldn't stay still. Life consisted of surviving his tics. For hours he'd sit with his back against the wall and slip his palm behind his head. When people called, Debra held the phone far away so he wouldn't smash his head against it—or her. At his worst he had to lie in bed with pillows lining each side so he wouldn't fall. If he had to go somewhere, he had to crawl.

This wasn't life—it was torture. And one way or another, he resolved to stop it.

With great difficulty, he marshaled his resolve to prepare for the meeting of his life. Exhausted and with bloodshot eyes, he studied Maciunas's credentials and managed to fill a half-inch black binder with research he had done over the last three years on Tourette's and deep brain stimulation. He included colorful PET scans of the brains of people with Tourette's, a description of his own tics, and a letter giving Maciunas permission to perform DBS that held him blameless, regardless of the outcome.

At the same time, he prepared his contingency plan, which consisted of the following three ways to end his life:

1. Lie down on nearby train tracks at night.
2. Take an overdose of mixed medications and household poisons.
3. Flood the garage with carbon monoxide from a running car.

The train tracks seemed like the best choice. He checked schedules to find out when trains crossed nearby tracks after dark. He envisioned how it would go. Dressed in black jeans, black hiking boots, and a black three-quarter-length leather jacket with matching leather gloves, he would lie on his stomach with his body perpendicular to the tracks. Then he would say his final prayers.

God, please forgive me for the action I am about to take. I hope you realize I have tried everything with the people and resources that you've provided me. I have loved, I have lived, and I have conquered more things than others can imagine in two lifetimes. I hope that you know and understand my reasons. Please let my family understand that it's too much for a human being to bear. I just want to be with you, God, as a guardian angel for my family and other families afflicted with other such diseases.

After lying down on the tracks he'd blast Guns N' Roses so loudly through his headphones he couldn't hear anything else. Then he'd turn his head away from the lights, rest his head on his extended arms, and wait for the train.

That was the easy part. The hard part would be looking his parents in the eye before he did it.

How can I tell them I love them, give them and a kiss and hug, and walk away knowing the next time they're going to see me it will be in

a casket? he thought. *How do I thank them for all that they have done*
for me? For raising me well and giving me a fun childhood filled with
memories? How do I do that to a mom and dad who not only told me that
they loved me but showed me every day? How do I do that to my only
brother, who has been my role model, my confidant, and right-hand man
and best friend?

Thinking about death was hard. But it had to be done.

Just in case.

Jeff never had life insurance. He didn't have any money. His most important possession was a cedar chest. He lifted the lid. Inside were letters of prayer and support from his grandparents and red-and-white crocheted Valentine's Day hearts from his grandmother.

He lifted one up that read "I love you, grandson," then set it back down.

The most meaningful things he kept in the trunk were a six-by-six-inch framed picture of St. Joseph that had been displayed in the casket at his Grandpa Matovic's wake and two of his grandpa's prayer books written in Slovak.

He closed the lid, then closed his eyes.

THE MORNING OF the meeting Jeff's mouth was dry and he could hear his heartbeat. He rehearsed his presentation in his mind, visualizing the scene and trying to think positively. His muscles were so hot from violent thrashing, he took an ice-cold shower. After he got out, he threw two ice packs around his shoulders and looked at himself in the mirror. Even after the cold shower, the ice bags melted quickly on the back of his hot neck.

"This man is going to understand," he said, staring into his own brown eyes. "He has to understand you, Jeff."

He stepped away to pace back and forth like tiger in a cage. Then he said out loud, "He's going to say yes today. He's got no choice!"

He continued icing his chest and his neck. Then he pointed at himself in the mirror. "You go do what you have to do," he said. "And get it done!" He pulled on a pair of blue North Carolina gym shorts, a short-sleeved white T-shirt, and a pair of white high-top Reeboks with dark blue trim.

TAKE A CHANCE ON ME

At University Hospitals Jeff was ushered into Maciunas's office and told the doctor would be with him in a moment. The office was standard issue, with pictures of the brain and nervous system on the wall and framed articles about movement disorders and neurosurgery.

As he waited for the doctor, Jeff played with a plastic model of a brain on the doctor's desk. Its four color-coded sections could be taken apart. As he held the right hemisphere of the brain, an explosive tic in his right arm caused him to spike the piece like a football. It slammed hard off the ground and went flying, bouncing off the exam table and hitting the wall. Mortified, Jeff scrambled around on his hand and knees to find it.

Oh, Lord! he thought. *Don't let him walk in now.* Ticking ferociously, he finally found the part by Maciunas's chair, wedged between the wall and the exam table. Quickly he put the model back together and made sure it was facing the right way. As he sat back down, sweat dripped into his eyes and ran down his nose.

Man! Jeff thought. *If he says yes, I certainly hope he takes better care of my brain than I did of that model!*

He turned around in time to see the doctor walk in the room. "You must be Jeff Matovic," Maciunas said with a genuine smile. "How are you today? I'm Dr. Maciunas. It's a pleasure to meet you."

The meeting lasted an hour and fifteen minutes. In it Jeff did his best to persuade Maciunas of three things: that his worsening Tourette's had boxed him into a corner, leaving him with a life that wasn't worth living; that he wasn't crazy, just in pain; and that he just knew that deep brain stimulation could be the answer he was looking for.

Maciunas felt the urgency in the visitor's voice and saw the passion in his eyes. He was awed by Jeff's intelligence, moved by his struggle, and impressed by his in-depth knowledge of the operation's risks and benefits. But he also knew Jeff was a true believer who had convinced himself that DBS was a panacea that would end his decades of unimaginable suffering. For Maciunas, that wasn't enough. He had to be sure that Jeff knew that the operation—while it had helped others with movement disorders—had no guarantee of helping him. In fact, he said, it had only been performed three times on patients with Tourette's—all of them in the Netherlands.

"And I have to tell you, Jeff, they were not completely successful," he said. Still, he was intrigued by the challenge and by the opportunity to change a life.

Finally, he came to a decision. "DBS looks like a viable option," he said. "But I can't promise you anything. I'll need about three weeks to see if you're a good candidate for the surgery." He wanted to do more research and have Jeff evaluated by several of his colleagues.

It wasn't a yes. But it wasn't a no.

"I'd like to start by having you meet with a colleague of mine," he said. "He's an excellent neurologist named Brian Maddux. If at any point any of this looks like it isn't fitting your needs, we will stop. But if it is fitting your needs, we will keep going. Does that sound good?"

"That sounds *great*," Jeff said. "Just *great*."

33

A Real Kick in the . . . Pants

LET'S GET THIS straight. Jeff never *tries* to kick his doctors in the crotch. Sometimes it just happens. In the fall of 2003 it happened during an examination with the good-natured neurologist named Brian Maddux at University Hospitals of Cleveland. Maddux was one of several "gatekeepers" Jeff had to get past if he had any hopes of being accepted for deep brain stimulation surgery.

Before the meeting Jeff glanced around the small office—exam table, X-ray machine, medical odds and ends. By far the most interesting thing in the room was the doctor.

Maddux bore little resemblance to the PermaPrest pretty boys you find on afternoon soaps. Tall, bearded, and rumpled, he had a mop of curly dark hair that seemed to go where it pleased. His tie was slightly off-center and loosened at the knot. Unlike most other doctors, he didn't wear a lab coat.

His uniform of choice was a short-sleeved shirt, even on the coldest winter days. But what he lacked in style he more than made up for in substance. He smiled when he met Jeff and quickly apologized for not looking more doctorlike. "I always feel like such a *geek* in a lab coat," he said.

Jeff liked him immediately. He tried to block his tics, or at least slow them down so he wouldn't look like a total goober. Maddux took out a blank notebook and a pen.

"Dr. Maddux, did you receive the information that I requested from the Cleveland Clinic?" Jeff asked in a halting voice, grunting and flailing his arms as he tried to steady himself in a chair.

"Yeah, we have it," Maddux said.

"Did you . . . look at it?"

"Nope. And I don't want to."

Jeff furrowed his brow.

"I need to get a clear picture of you," Maddux continued. "And I need to get it from ground level."

Jeff writhed as if trying wriggle out of a strait jacket. He was breathing hard, and streams of perspiration ran down his flushed face. As he talked, Maddux stopped him several times to hand him cooling drinks of water. "Did you . . . thank you," Jeff said, stopping to sip some water. "Did you read over my notes when I met with Dr. Maciunas?"

"No," said Maddux.

"Don't you think you might want to?"

Maddux put his hand on Jeff's bouncing shoulder. "Relax," he said in a reassuring voice. "We work well as a team. I need to get the neurological picture of you. But I can't do that if I have a biased scene in front of me."

At Maddux's direction Jeff moved from his chair to the exam table, a cold, padded, rectangular bench that seemed to be swathed in butcher paper. Even at Jeff's height, his feet did not touch the ground. His tennis shoes swung nervously back and forth at the end of his long legs.

Leaning in, Maddux began the standard neurological workup. He wanted to examine Jeff's ears and eyes with a light and have him touch his fingers to his nose. Easier said than done. Jeff flopped like a fish out of water, pulling away each time the doctor got close. For Maddux, the examination quickly became an exercise in patience. For Jeff, it was just another in a long line of embarrassing moments.

"Dr. Maddux, I am *so* sorry," he said in a voice that was as contrite as it was mortified.

"Perfectly OK," Maddux said. "I want you to feel like there's nothing you need to hold back." The words comforted Jeff. He liked everything about Dr. Maddux. He made him feel safe, like there was nothing he had to hide.

So he didn't—and his tics exploded! As if waging a small war against the examination, the Tourette's made him swing his arms wildly. Suddenly he was a drunken boxer, flailing and thrashing wildly, striking Maddux with a dizzying combination of blows.

Oh, God, he thought. *What an impression to make on my new doctor!*

Again, Maddux reassured him with an it's-all-right smile. "If you don't feel free to tic in my office, I can't get a good picture of you," he said, moving back and doing his best to ignore the unintentional onslaught.

But it *was* easier to do an examination when you weren't getting pummeled like a heavy bag. Jeff agreed to sit on his hands in an effort to limit the assault.

Maddux moved to Jeff's right side and resumed his efforts to take a look in his ear. Placing his thigh against Jeff's knee, he physically held his head still with his left hand.

He's a saint, Jeff thought. *As badly as I'm ticking, he's making it seem like it's no big deal.*

"Jeff," Maddux said. "I'm going to have to hold you kind of tight to hold you still," he said. "When you feel the pressure cooker about to blow, you let me know. In between, I'll try to get a look." With Jeff taking deep breaths in between heavy tics, Maddux successfully examined both ears.

"Now I want to take a look at your eyes," he said.

Oh, this ought to be fun, Jeff thought.

Not only was he blinking about a hundred times a minute, his head was moving like a bobblehead doll's—a six-foot-five bobblehead doll with a head the size of a bowling ball.

"Jeff," Maddux said. "I want you to stare at a spot on the wall."

"Which wall?" Jeff said, trying to focus through the tics.

"The dot on this wall that I'm tapping," Maddux said, tap-tap-tapping the spot on the wall.

Jeff's spoke in halting and broken tones as he did his best to turn his unsteady head to try to find the spot. He was sweating. Exhausted. Determined.

"OK," he said. "I hear . . . you tapping." His neck wrenched violently as his body rejected any notion of control. "I can't . . ." he grunted and forced air out of his lungs loudly. "Wait," he said. "I'll find it."

He finally located the spot on the wall. "Let me take a couple of deep breaths, and get some water to cool my face down," he said.

While he breathed, Maddux approached him from the front. Unable to get close, he shone his penlight in Jeff's eye from about a foot away. Afterward, he dimmed the lights in the room. The dark was comforting.

Maddux approached again, this time standing directly in front of Jeff in the darkened room. "Now I'm going to have to get *this close* to you," he said, indicating several inches with his fingers.

HEAD BUTT! Jeff thought.

It wasn't like he'd ever *try* to head butt anyone, least of all Dr. Maddux, a compassionate doctor trying to help him. But things just had a way of happening when people got too close. "Dr. Maddux," Jeff stammered. "I'm not sure you want to do that. Because if I jerk my head I don't want to hurt you."

He was more than capable of hurting him. Jeff was not only tall, but bull strong. He was cut, his muscles hyperdeveloped from years of violent and constant ticking, which was better than any workout you could get in a gym. Another doctor once figured that his constant ticking was the equivalent of doing more than eighty thousand crunches in a twenty-four-hour period.

Maddux just smiled. "I've been kicked, hit, head butted, bitten. Honestly, as long as you don't send me to my own emergency room, I'm OK with that."

Jeff laughed and a bit of the tension eased from his body. He took several deep breaths as Maddux moved in slowly and got a good look at Jeff's right eye. He moved swiftly to the left eye, trying to take advantage of a rare calm moment.

Jeff usually felt the pressure boiling inside of him whenever a huge tic was coming. Not this time. With Maddux looking in his left eye, Jeff's swinging right leg unleashed a savage kick, hitting Maddux square in the groin. Maddux flashed an uncomfortable smile. If it hurt, he never said so.

"I got a good look," he said, moving away gingerly. "Let's get something to drink and sit down and talk."

34

Testing, Testing

ONE GATEKEEPER DOWN, one to go.

To make sure Jeff was a good candidate for DBS surgery, Dr. Robert Maciunas enlisted the help of a neuropsychologist named Dr. Paula O'Grocki. Her job: put Jeff through a six-hour battery of complex psychological, gross motor, and intelligence tests.

O'Grocki needed to know what percentage of each hemisphere of his brain Jeff used. If he was either too left-brained or too right-brained, the operation might pose too great a risk or just not work. If Jeff wanted to have deep brain stimulation, this was one exam he couldn't fail.

The tests took place in September 2003 at a University Hospitals' satellite branch in a large space that reminded Jeff of a living room. It had two area rugs, pictures on the wall, live plants, and an L-shaped wooden desk lit by dappled sunlight.

After Jeff entered the room, Dr. O'Grocki welcomed him with a warm smile and a pleasant greeting that made him feel he was in good hands.

"Is there anything in particular in the room that bothers you in any way?" she said. "Are there any pictures you don't like? Is the lighting OK? Too bright? Too dim?"

A scented candle sat nearby. "Can you smell the candle?" she said.

"Yes," Jeff said, sensing a fresh fragrance that smelled like ocean mist.

"Does it smell good to you?"

"Yes."

Jeff sat in a hard-backed plastic chair as the questions kept coming.

"Are you comfortable in the chair?" "Are you sure?" "How are you feeling today?" "Is there anything else you need?"

It was O'Grocki's job to make sure Jeff was at ease and that absolutely nothing skewed the tests.

"I'm fine, really," Jeff assured her.

The doctor explained the order and types of tests he would be given and the importance of each. For a psychology major like Jeff, it was fascinating. There were short- and long-term memory tests, dexterity tests, reading retention tests, fine and gross motor movement tests. She had him put pegs in holes and do logic puzzles. Some of the tests were done with both hands, others with the right or the left alone. Many were timed. In one test she asked him to name any word that began with the letter *S* and then said "Go!"

"Uh . . . saw, sing, salmon, soup," Jeff said. "Slime. Slimy. Silly. Sentry. Umm. Sanitation. S-sss-saxophone. Sick. Saturday. Singular. Sangria. Sanctimonious." Jeff raced through the *S*-words in his head as his Tourette's made him flex, punch, and kick.

The logic puzzles were next. Leaning forward in his chair, he fit all the wooden pieces together. Then he moved on to plastic and metal puzzles with abstract designs, solving each of them just as fast.

He laughed. This was one test where his OCD came in handy. It helped him recognize shapes and angles and patterns. "Done," Jeff said, snapping the last puzzle piece into place.

"Wow!" O'Grocki said, surprised he had finished so quickly.

In a cognitive memory test, Jeff was given paper and a pencil. O'Grocki then held up a drawing with a variety of abstract designs for Jeff to study for ten seconds. Then she put the picture down.

"Ready, set, go," she said. Jeff's job was to recreate as much of the picture, by drawing, as he could.

In another test of both short- and long-term memory, she read Jeff a short story. An hour later, after Jeff had undergone a variety of other tests, she looked at her patient.

"Do you remember the story I read you?" she asked.

"Yes," Jeff said.

"I'm going to ask you some basic questions that pertain to that story." The questions ranged from recalling a character's name or a destination to something more abstract, such as the moral of the story. She had him recall colors, such as a red schoolhouse a character walked by, as well as familial relationships, ages, and other details.

"It will take several weeks to fully interpret these tests, write out my report, and then discuss it with Dr. Maciunas," O'Grocki said.

"Dr. O'Grocki," Jeff said. "I'm at my boiling point. I have to know your initial thoughts."

She smiled. "Not only are you going to have my full recommendation for the procedure, I couldn't have handpicked a better candidate." Jeff let out a huge sigh.

Several weeks later, Jeff and Debra met again with Maciunas in his office.

"Well, I've got some news," he told the couple, as they held hands and hung on his every word.

"And?" Jeff said.

"We've got final approval," Maciunas said. "We're going to do the operation."

Jeff bent over and sobbed openly into his hands, gulping his breaths in gasps.

"Thank you so much!" he said through his tears in a trembling voice.

"You're very welcome," Maciunas said.

Jeff's arm shot out from the side of his body, and his leg kicked the front of Maciunas's wooden desk so hard it made it move.

This was what he had been praying for. He still had tics, but now he had something else: hope. He blinked back tears as he stood up and embraced Maciunas. After the meeting he stopped three times to cry on his way out of the hospital.

It was another hurdle cleared. But it was far from the last or the highest one. The operation cost a quarter million dollars—and he had no insurance.

That was bad.

What was worse was that even if he did have insurance, deep brain stimulation was not FDA-approved for Tourette's. That meant there was a good chance an insurance company would deny coverage. That wasn't a hurdle as much as a giant stone wall. Without insurance approval, Jeff would have to find a way to raise $250,000 or work with the hospital to get grants. That could take years, if it even worked at all.

But maybe there was a way. Maciunas was truthful but vague on insurance forms. He wrote "DBS for a movement disorder" instead of "DBS for Tourette's." If the insurance company didn't ask *which* movement disorder, Maciunas wasn't about to tell.

It was a chance they needed to take. But first Jeff needed to get on Debra's insurance plan—now. They knew what they had to do. They scrapped their dream wedding at the Renaissance Fair for a simple ceremony at Lyndhurst City Hall. They got the license, and in three weeks they were married. Jeff's tics relented enough to let him enjoy the moment with his bride. After the hugs and the kisses, the smiles and the handshakes, Debra added Jeff to her insurance. Then they both held their breath as they sought preapproval for coverage of Jeff's costly surgery.

35

Quarter-Million-Dollar Insurance Dance

JEFF COULD HARDLY walk. But now he had to run.

Grunting, twitching, blinking, punching, head shaking, arms flailing, he dropped his cell phone and began doing laps around his living room. Jubilant but unsteady, he raced through the place like a lush who'd hit the lottery. Socks slipping on hardwood floor, he fell down, jumped up, and pawed pictures off the wall. As he crashed into couches and knocked knickknacks to the floor, his four cats scattered as if running from a Rottweiler.

"Yes!" he screamed, pumping his fists between spastic shakes and spectacular crashes. "Yes! Yes!"

Bruises? Broken furniture? He didn't care. He was finally getting the one thing that had eluded him for more than three decades.

A chance to be normal.

The insurance agent had just called with the news of whether the company was going to cover the cost of the quarter-million-dollar brain surgery that just possibly could save his life. He had been waiting for the call for what seemed like years, praying for a good outcome. When it finally came time, he couldn't breathe.

This is it, he thought after the caller identified himself. *If we don't get this, we'll have to wait, try to get a grant, or have fund-raisers.* A no easily could have delayed everything for five years or more. He couldn't wait five years.

Then he heard the voice on the other end. "Mister Matovic?" It was dull, bland, and utterly devoid of any personality or spark.

Oh, no, he thought. *It's bad news. Nobody can be that dull if it's good news.* And yet . . .

"I want to give you a confirmation code," the man said in a buttoned-down monotone.

"Confirmation code?" Jeff said. "What does a confirmation code mean?"

"Mr. Matovic," said the voice, slow as a Sunday sermon. "Your insurance is going to cover your procedure. Your appointment with Dr. Maciunas is scheduled for November eleventh."

That's it! It happened!

Nearly vibrating with excitement, he clambered clumsily from the living room into the great room and back again, stopping only briefly when he ran into something or fell over.

"Ahhhhh!" he yelled, waving his arms. "Thank you, Gaaahhhdddd!"

And yet crying out wasn't enough—he had to run, he had to jump, he had to . . . *dance*! After twenty frantic laps he finally stopped long enough to call Debra at work. But when she answered he was so emotional all he could do was blubber into the receiver.

"Oh, honey, it's OK," Debra said in a brave voice, assuming the worst. "We'll find a way."

Then Jeff found his voice. "Babe," he said, breathing hard, and with trembles of emotion in his voice, "how would you like your day to get a whole helluva lot better?"

"Tell me, babe!" Debra said, her mood brightening.

"We're approved!" Jeff shouted.

"Ahhhhhhhhhhhhh!" Debra screamed, jumping to her feet in her office. It was almost too much to process. It was everything they had ever wanted. They had hope. They had a yes from one of the top neurosurgeons in the country. And now they had insurance approval!

If the operation ended up working, Jeff knew he'd have to thank his doctors. But there was someone else vitally important to all of this whom he didn't know he'd have to thank.

Frankenstein.

36

The Story of Medtronic

IN 1932 EARL Bakken—the man who would start the company that made the stimulators doctors planned to put in Jeff's brain—was an eight-year-old boy growing up in the Minneapolis suburb of Columbia Heights. Young Earl had always been fascinated with electricity. But one Saturday afternoon at the Heights Theater on Central Avenue, he saw a movie that took that interest in a whole new direction.

Frankenstein.

Written by Mary Wollstonecraft Shelley—wife of English romantic poet Percy Bysshe Shelley—when she was only twenty-one, *Frankenstein* told the story of a "mad" scientist who used electricity to bring to life a creature made from salvaged body parts. In the 1931 film adaptation, director James Whale used high-arcing transformers to dramatically show the power of electrical energy flowing into the creature's body. As he sat through the movie again and again, young Earl was fascinated by the restorative properties of Dr. Frankenstein's life-giving electricity.

Inspired, the imaginative third-grader began dreaming of building actual stimulation devices that would restore life—or help keep people alive. He conducted his own experiments with electricity in the basement workshop of his boyhood home. As he grew, Bakken continued his interest in futuristic medical electricity. He carried that interest to the University of Minnesota, where he studied electrical engineering in graduate school. His interest in the evolving field of medical electricity often prompted him to visit the university's new biomedical school, where teachers and their students were merging medical technology with engineering technology. He met fascinating people there who worked with electrocardiograms and other electrical devices in clinical labs.

In 1949 hospitals, clinics, and academic labs had just started to use some of the electronics developed in World War II. The problem: they had no one to fix the machines when they broke. Knowing Bakken was a graduate student in electrical engineering, professors at the biomedical school asked him if he could repair some of their broken medical equipment.

He jumped at chance. Suddenly Bakken was eight years old again, sitting in the Heights Theater on Central Avenue watching Dr. Frankenstein infuse the monster with life-giving electricity. Learning by doing, he repaired EKG machines, flame photometers, osmometers, and pH meters.

Later, at a family birthday party he told his brother-in-law, Palmer Hermundslie, what he had been doing. That gave Hermundslie an idea. "Maybe there's a business in setting up a quality repair service for medical electronic equipment," he said.

They didn't analyze the idea or study its market potential. Bakken simply quit graduate school and Hermundslie gave up his job at a lumberyard. On April 9, 1949, they started their business, which they called Medtronic, out of a garage.

From the beginning, Bakken employed a philosophy he called "Ready, Fire, Aim!" That full-speed-ahead philosophy allowed him to honor innovation over more practical considerations, such as money and market. Bakken wasn't interested in limitations, only possibilities.

There were many struggles along the way that would have caused lesser men to quit. But with Bakken's talents, and a lot of Hermundslie's money, they rode out the lean years. Despite occasionally teetering on the brink of bankruptcy, their visions began to become reality.

In 1957, eight years after founding the company, they had their first breakthrough. Bakken invented the battery-operated, transistorized, wearable artificial pacemaker, the first of many advancements that turned Medtronic into a global leader.

As Medtronic grew, Bakken urged employees not to limit themselves and motivated them to think in unstructured ways to chase the impossible dream. His approach helped employees to be fearless and to "break the bonds of excessive caution and crippling self-restraint." Bakken encouraged his employees to follow their hunches, no matter how far-fetched or seemingly impractical. Bakken once said to an interviewer: "Most of the good things in my life and career have come to pass because somebody was willing to rush in where more careful folks were afraid to tread."

Bakken and his team created many useful technological products for the body, including radio frequency therapies, various mechanical devices, drug and biologic delivery systems, and diagnostic tools used to treat more than thirty chronic diseases. His company now employs forty thousand people, has annual revenues in excess of $14 billion (2009 figures) and has helped millions of patients in more than 120 countries.

Bakken, who many consider an engineering genius, won such prestigious honors as the National Academy of Engineering's Rust Prize and the IEEE Centennial Medal. He is widely credited with creating the medical device industry. But even a brilliant medical device is useless without an equally brilliant neurosurgeon who knows where to put it and how to make it work.

37

Dr. Robert J. Maciunas

EVERY YEAR ON his birthday—March 15—Robert Maciunas picked up the telephone at exactly 12:24 PM and called his mother to thank her for giving birth to him. He called her when he was in medical school. He called her after he got married. He kept calling her, year after year, even after he became an internationally respected neurosurgeon. If he didn't have the time, he *made* the time. Some things were just too important to let slip, and appreciation for his mother topped the list.

Above all, Maciunas was a family man with a caring heart as large as his towering intellect. Which is why, on his first birthday after his mother died, when he realized he could no longer make his yearly call, he sat down and he cried.

As a group, neurosurgeons can be an arrogant lot. Brash. Conceited. Self-important. Sensitivity is not part of the job description. They do better with audacity, like an NFL quarterback or an air force fighter pilot.

Bob Maciunas was a notable exception. A renaissance man who loved art and history as much as midbrains and microsurgery, he cared deeply about the feelings of others. He read poetry and wrote love sonnets to his wife, worked in homeless shelters, and taught his sons, Nick and Joe, the importance of simple human decency.

"Dad always taught me to be respectful of everyone," said Nick, his oldest. "Not just people with authority, or those who might help me out in the future. He always made a point of saying hello and thank you to janitors, even when we were just passing through a place. . . . It was very important to him to make sure that people were appreciated for their work, no matter how small the task. He was kind in many ways, but this simple generosity particularly stood out to me."

His skill as a surgeon stood out as well. Consistently recognized by his peers, Maciunas was one of the best neurosurgeons in the world. By his early fifties he had written 106 peer-reviewed journal articles, nine books, and thirty-one chapters in the books of others. He had given more than three hundred conference presentations and held ten patents. An expert in deep brain stimulation who liked to use his creativity to find novel solutions to complex problems, he once called his work "an equal mix of high science and high art."

Medical skill ran deep in his Lithuanian roots. His mother, Genevive, was a dentist. His father, Algirdas, was chair of general surgery at Vytautas Didysis University in Kaunas, Lithuania, while his grandfather served as the country's minister of health.

When the KGB entered Lithuania in the 1940s, his parents fled to the United States with their three daughters. Bob was born in Chicago and grew up wanting to be a doctor. In 1976, at the age of twenty-one, he graduated from Northwestern University with a bachelor's in biochemistry. After completing his studies in 1980 at Abraham Lincoln School of Medicine at the University of Illinois, he did his residency at the Mayo Clinic, learning both general surgery and neurosurgery.

The Mayo Clinic gave him something else too—his future wife, Ann Failinger. Ann worked as a neurology and neurosurgical social worker. She often helped Maciunas's patients who needed counseling or special care after leaving the hospital. One of them was an eighty-four-year-old woman who recently had become Miss Gray Panther of Minnesota.

"You're going to marry my doctor one day," she said. "He would be *perfect* for you." Ann smiled and nodded. But she hadn't even met Bob Maciunas.

That soon changed. A week later he saw her walking down the hall and declared for himself: "That's the woman I'm going to marry one day." Not long after, in 1983, the predictions came true. On a frigid day in Rochester, Minnesota, Robert Maciunas and Ann Failinger married in St. Mary's Chapel inside the Mayo Clinic.

One day Ann, still working as a medical social worker, showed an interest in medicine while working beside a doctor. "It was fun to try to figure out the diagnosis," she said.

"You should go to medical school!" her husband said.

"You're nuts," she said with a laugh. Ann didn't believe she was smart enough. It didn't matter. Bob Maciunas saw potential, and he moved quickly to encourage it.

"I'm going to lock this door," he said, gently shooing his wife out of the house. "Don't come back until you've signed up for pre-med courses."

She enrolled and took the courses. Eight years later, after moving to Nashville and having a son, she graduated from Vanderbilt Medical School and became a pediatrician.

Ann still could not believe what her husband had inspired her to do after the couple moved to suburban Cleveland, where he took a job at Case Western Reserve University School of Medicine—and later, with University Hospitals of Cleveland. But then Bob Maciunas believed in people, often more than they believed in themselves. He pushed and prodded, nudged and encouraged. Instead of coming up with a thousand reasons why they couldn't do something, he urged them to find one reason why they could.

In Maciunas's world, nothing was impossible with enough work, passion, and love. His was a world filled with beauty. He seemed to absorb art and poetry straight through his skin. He treasured good wine, good coffee, classical music, and classic rock—and spoke Lithuanian, German, Spanish, and a little Russian. He seemed to know everything about everything. A fellow physician once said he had "the biggest hard drive" of anyone he had ever known.

But of all the passions in his life, his greatest love was reserved for his family. He cared deeply about his boys' education, helping them with difficult homework and encouraging them to stretch themselves academically.

From their family home in Chagrin Falls, Ohio, he and Ann traveled extensively with the boys, taking them to Europe to show them the world's great works of art and to Alaska and the Rocky Mountains to see nature's splendor. During their trips he regaled his boys with detailed facts, wanting them not just to see the sights but to appreciate the history, culture, food, language, politics, and geography.

Above all, he wanted his sons to develop character.

By all accounts, they did. Nick and Joe both played on a soccer team for Hawken, the private school they attended. One day, after Joe had a rough day in goal, he handled it with grace. Afterward Maciunas told a friend, Oberlin College dance professor and choreographer Carter McAdams, that he couldn't have been prouder of Joe than if he had made the winning save.

"It's so incredible to be a father and watch your son become a man right in front of your eyes," he said. Despite a busy schedule, Maciunas did his best to make all of his sons' soccer games, including the Ohio state championship in 2005. The game before, Nick had helped score the winning goal, sending Hawken to the finals.

"Oh my God," Maciunas said, realizing he had a conflict. "What am I going to do?"

He had to fly to Germany to give a speech at a prestigious international neurosurgical conference the day before the championship game. Other people would have made their apologies and missed the finals. Not Bob Maciunas. He left on a Wednesday evening and flew overnight to Germany. On Thursday he gave a fifteen-minute speech, then rushed back to the airport and flew nine hours home to make the game.

Hawken lost. But to Maciunas, that wasn't the point. You cared deeply. You gave it your all. You found a way. *That* was the point.

And so it was with his patients. When Jeff Matovic poured out his heart to Robert Joseph Maciunas, he did not do so in vain. After years of frustration with other doctors, his pleas had finally reached someone who cared deeply, someone who would give it his all, someone who would find a way.

Maciunas was struck by Jeff's resilience and bravery and deeply moved by his struggle. He saw him not just as a patient or a problem, but as a human being. When he got home that night he poured himself a glass of wine and sat with his wife on a love seat in their long kitchen. Ann had never seen her husband so eager to tell a story. He looked at her with tears in his eyes.

"I saw a patient today who just broke my heart," he said, describing Jeff's collection of painful tics. "How could he live this way for as long as he has? How could he maintain any sense of dignity or sanity? I want to help this guy. I really want to help this guy!"

Maciunas talked about how thin Jeff looked. "He burns off more calories in five minutes that I do in two weeks!"

He talked about how Jeff was willing to put his life on the line. "I can't believe how brave he is," he said. "I could *never* do that!"

Over the next several months he became obsessed with Jeff's case, spending many sleepless nights reading up on similar surgeries around the world, none of which had been completely successful. Night after night he called Brian Maddux and other physicians to brainstorm, applying everything he knew to the available medical literature. In between he prayed—at St. Paul's Episcopal in Cleveland Heights and at home. "We need God's help to heal," he told his wife.

"Bob," his wife told him, "you've been blessed with a wonderful set of hands. God will be with you in that surgery. He sees your intentions to change Jeff's life. He will help you."

The night before the surgery, Bob Maciunas was restless. He brought five neurosurgery books and eighteen journal articles that he had laid on out the kitchen table to the couple's king-sized bed.

"I just want to make it better for him," he said, his eyes darting between the books as if cramming for a final exam. "I just want to make it *better.*"

Ann had never seen her husband this anxious. "Honey," she finally said. "You're not going to make it better unless you shut up and go sleep. Let's just sit and relax."

She rubbed his back until he finally fell asleep.

38

Keep Calm

THE PHONE RANG many times in the months before the surgery. Mostly it was family and friends asking about Jeff. Switching her gaze between her husband and the ringing phone, Debra would hold up her hand as if to say "I got it." Her job: give them the information, run interference, shoo them away.

Jeff couldn't talk to them anyway. With the severity of his tics, his words would be gibberish, peppered with forced exhalations of air. Besides, his arm tics might cause him to whack himself on the side of the head with the phone.

Debra always repeated what the caller said so that Jeff could hear. Their sentiments were nice. But so many people called that it got old after awhile. Eventually she started making jokes.

"How's Jeff doing?" she repeated, smiling and winking at Jeff. "Oh, you know, he's just typing out the eighty-fifth page of his PhD dissertation on particle physics," she said. "He's presenting it tomorrow to the board."

But callers couldn't help but hear his explosive verbal tics in the background.

"Huh-*HUHHHHH*!"

"Don't worry," Debra said. "He's just swinging an aluminum bat. He's playing catch outside in the backyard with Mike."

"*HUH!* I really got a hold of that one," Jeff would yell.

Then she'd smile, thank them for their kindness, and tell them that everything was going as well as could be expected.

As Jeff waited for his surgery, he had to remain as calm as he could. No unnecessary stress or stimulation of any kind. Doctors' orders. They had one shot at this, and they didn't want to take any chances. Jeff wasn't to take phone calls or go to parties. He even had to bow out of his family's annual Christmas celebration.

Not all of his friends or family understood. And why would they? Jeff hadn't told them everything. He hadn't told them how risky the operation was or that it could kill him. He just didn't want them to worry or, worse, try to talk him out of it. His mind was made up.

In the months before the operation, Jeff ate more fruits and vegetables than he had in his life. He walked with extra care, washed his hands excessively, avoided germs at all costs, held on to things when he could. He just didn't want to get sick, injure himself, or do anything that could compromise the surgery. He was in full protection mode. He almost wanted to surround himself with bumper rails or live inside a bubble.

Then it happened. Debra heard a loud bang as Jeff crumpled to the floor. "Oh my God," she said. While walking through the dining room Jeff's body shook violently from head to toe, as hard as it had in several months. He lost his balance and fell, slamming his head hard enough against the dining room wall to put a dent in it and wake up the kids upstairs.

"You're going to be OK," Debra said, sitting on the floor, rocking and holding Jeff tightly as a tear rolled slowly down her cheek. "You're going to be OK. You're going to be OK. Remember, you're a *tough* one."

Jeff nodded his head.

"It's going to take more than this to stop you."

Jeff nodded and squeezed her hand.

"You hear me?"

He nodded.

"All right," she said, stroking his arm. "OK. It's all right. It's all right." Debra looked at the dent in the dining room wall and smiled. "You got a damn hard head, you know that?"

39

Last Rites

THREE WEEKS BEFORE the surgery, Jeff came to his parents with a request. He asked them to say a prayer, asking God if the surgery was not going to be successful to simply let him die on the table.

Jeff *had* to believe the operation was going to work. But he also had to be realistic. This was major brain surgery, and one of its risks was death. No matter what happened, he needed to be prepared—just in case. He asked a priest to give him last rites.

One week before the operation, accompanied only by his father, he attended an intimate Mass in a small section of St. Francis Chapel used for baptisms and special blessings. For Jeff, getting last rites was a spiritual and mental housecleaning, a way to prepare and bless his body for God should something go wrong on the operating table.

Jeff wanted the blessing. What he *did not* want was a circus, with dozens of friends and family blubbering over him and making a scene. This was too personal. This was between him and his God.

The Mass, conducted by Father Casey Bukala, a balding priest in his early seventies with kind eyes and a light brown moustache, began at 5:30 PM. Jeff had requested an evening mass because he loved how the sun shone through a breathtaking circle of stained glass in the back of the chapel. During the service Jeff asked for forgiveness for his sins.

"God," he prayed silently. "I know we've had our ups and downs. I've shut you out, I've held you close, and I've cursed your name. We've seen the ultimate highs and the ultimate lows. But I ask that with your forgiveness we will one day be able to see eye to eye."

In the middle of the Mass, Father Bukala called Jeff to the front for the blessing. As he faced the priest, Jeff suddenly had an overwhelming feeling of peace, and a sense that God's will would be done.

Jeff repeated the Lord's Prayer after the priest. Then Father Bukala brought out the holy oil in a crystal decanter. He took the lid off and dabbed his right thumb into the oil, which had been blessed before the service, and used it to make the sign of the cross on Jeff's forehead.

"Jeff," he said, "receive this special blessing of the Holy Spirit, and may peace find you and relieve you from your ailments so that you can be always one with the Lord." After, Father Bukala made the sign of the cross while facing Jeff and said, "In the name of the Father, the Son, and the Holy Spirit. May you receive this blessing."

"Amen," Jeff said. As he walked slowly back to his chair, he looked at his father and began to tremble. Would this be the last time he'd attend Mass with his dad? He closed his eyes and fell into his father's firm embrace.

"I love you," his father said, holding Jeff firmly while softly patting his back. "You're in God's hands now. He'll guide you to wherever you need to be. I'm so proud of you for becoming the man that you are, and for all that you've overcome."

40

Tic Tic Tic

JEFF TWITCHED. HE couldn't have twitched harder if he had been struck by lightning. Fighting for balance, he lurched across his living room. He took large steps, followed by short ones. Forward ones, followed by backward ones. His shoulders heaved, and his long arms flew out as if yanked by wires. Just before reaching the couch he crumpled to the floor.

In hours, surgeons would bore two holes in his head and peer deeply into the recesses of his brain. Late in the evening, an icy wind swirled outside his Cleveland suburb, and snow covered the street like a satin sheet. But inside, Jeff looked like he'd just stepped from a sauna. Rivers of sweat snaked down his bare chest. Alone in the darkness, he focused on a single thought: "Just make it to 4:00 AM."

Things would be better then. He looked at the clock. The shaking of his closely shaven head made the numbers dance and blur. 10:00 PM.

In a perfect world he might have passed the time with a TV show or book, a sandwich or a long run. Not on this night. Doctors had warned him not to have anything to eat or drink. He couldn't read for fear he'd rip the pages out of the book. TV would only activate his obsessive-compulsive disorder.

As for running? He couldn't even walk down the stairs. The only thing left: suffer. He curled into a ball as the nerve-jangling urges exploded across his body again, leaving him to writhe on the hardwood floor. He shifted in place, searching for a position that would satisfy the greedy compulsions. When he didn't find one, they shook him like a wet dog. His life wasn't so much about living anymore as surviving. But on this night, he told himself, that was enough—at least until 4:00 AM. It was a finish line of sorts. Or was it a starting line? Either way it was everything he had ever dreamed of, the answer to his prayers, the key to a new life—provided it didn't kill him first.

Four AM was when his alarm would ring, and he would head to the hospital. There, a team of specialists would root around in his brain while he was still awake, using an operation not approved for Tourette Syndrome, to do what they could to relieve a lifetime of suffering. His heart hammered in his chest. He wondered if this might be the last time he'd see his wife, Debra, or her children, Bonnie and Mike. He worried this might be the last time he'd talk to his mother and father, or his older brother, Steve.

Eleven thirty. His muscles burned. He was tired of ticking. Tired of worrying. Tired of waiting. Whatever the surgery would bring, he just wanted it to begin.

It would have been easier if he could have slept. He had tried. But when violent full-body spasms caused him to bounce off the bed like a trampoline artist, he gave up. Debra never complained. But Jeff knew she was just being nice.

He got up to go downstairs. *At least somebody should get some sleep,* he thought.

As he walked, the floorboards creaked beneath his toes, which had taken to thrusting him upward every few steps as if he were a gigantic ballerina. At the top of the stairs his arm flew out, then his leg. He grabbed the wooden handrail to keep himself from falling. He put a death grip on the railing as he started unsteadily down the first stair. Just then a powerful arm tic nearly caused him to rip the railing from the wall.

OK, he thought. *Maybe walking down the stairs by myself wasn't such a good idea.* He sat on the top step and bumped down the stairs on his bottom like a four-year-old. He felt silly, but it was better than breaking his neck. In the living room he sat on the glossy hardwood floor and tried to relax. But with the operation of his life scant hours away, his excitement pushed his tics to new levels.

A thin, cut athlete, Jeff was in superior shape. But he would have traded bodies with the Pillsbury Doughboy if it meant no more tics.

During a rare calm moment he leaned against the couch and fanned his hand across the top of his bristly black hair. His fingers pressed through his scalp to the hardness of his skull. He stopped at a familiar place on the crown of his head, and a chill ran through him.

This was where they were going to drill.

Adrenaline swept through his chest, and he punched his arm so hard his elbow cracked. "*HUH-HUH!*" he grunted, forcing air hard out of his mouth. He closed his eyes and said a prayer as the clock struck midnight.

He had almost made it. There would be no more "enduring" his Tourette's. After thirty-one years in hell he had reached a crossroads. Either he was going to get better, or he was going to die—even if it had to be by his own hand. He had committed to taking life pass-fail; his final exam was less than twelve hours away.

Twelve hours! he thought. It couldn't come quickly enough. If only he could watch TV.

He didn't dare. While his physical tics were hard to deal with, his mental tics could be even worse. When activated, they'd hold his brain hostage, looking for angles, calculating midpoints, fanatically multi-plying and dividing prime numbers like a malfunctioning computer. Recently he had watched a professional basketball game. His obsessive-compulsive disorder made him catalog everything from the bounces of the ball to the number of rotations it made on a shot. He knew it was stupid, fruitless. He also knew he couldn't stop it.

He passed the time by ticking and thinking about the operation. *They're going to be in my brain today,* he thought, smoothing his hand over the crown of his throbbing head. *And they're going to make it right.*

He looked at the clock again—3:47 AM. His father-in-law, Mike, would arrive soon to take them to the hospital. Most people called Mike "Doc." He'd come by the name honestly, having worked for decades as a podiatrist. Debra's parents lived two miles away. Doc volunteered to drive. Bonnie and Mike spent the night at their house.

Four AM. The alarm clock rang upstairs. Debra got out of bed, pulled on a robe, and walked downstairs to check on Jeff. She found him sitting on the floor, ticking hard and leaning against the couch.

"How long have you been there?"

"All . . . night," he said, barely getting the words out. "I—HUH! I thought it would be better to come down here so . . . I . . . wouldn't wake you, and you could get some . . . sleep."

"That's really sweet," Debra said. "But you didn't have to do that."

He tried to respond. She placed her index finger on his mouth. "Don't talk anymore. Your stuff's all packed."

She headed upstairs but stopped to glance back at her husband. Catching his eye, she walked back down and rubbed his shaved head, knowing his future—and hers—lay somewhere inside of it. They laughed, and he flashed a smile—that wide, goofy, irresistible smile that always made everything else about him disappear.

She bent toward him and placed both hands out as a protective barrier to keep an ill-timed shake from knocking out her teeth. Then, slowly, carefully, she kissed him on top of his head. "I'm going to go get my shower," she said. "You just relax."

Jeff climbed onto the couch and looked down the block in the pre-dawn darkness. A light snow fell. Some of the houses still had their Christmas lights on. *What a beautiful a day to go get my life back*, he thought.

Debra had packed for him the day before. The suitcase sat by the front door. Doc's minivan pulled into the driveway around 5:00 AM.

Grabbing him tightly so he wouldn't fall, Debra helped her husband into the seat behind hers and buckled him in. During the twenty-minute ride to the hospital, Jeff felt a strange feeling that he had rarely felt in the last few years—a feeling of control returning to his body and a sense of peace.

Looking out the back window he saw the tire tracks the van made in the snow. They made him think of his life—where he'd been and the places he was going. Shortly before 5:30, Doc pulled the van onto Euclid Avenue, then into the hospital's curving driveway. Debra helped Jeff out of the van. "Let's get you inside," she said. "It's cold."

"Deb," Jeff said, now able to speak. "Let me just stand here and feel this. It's going to be a few days before I'm able to get fresh air again."

He faced the hospital doors, sucking in as much of the cold air as his lungs would hold. He glanced back down Euclid Avenue. For a moment, he froze, not moving, thinking about everything and nothing at the same time. He thought again about his life as the sparkling snow danced and swirled in the whipping winter wind. He took a few last deep breaths, promising to remember how good they had felt.

Finally ready, he turned back to Debra. "All right," he said, "let's go."

41

The Pre-Op Comedy Hour

University Hospitals, Cleveland, Ohio. February 9, 2004.

On an excitement scale, waiting for surgery alone in a tiny hospital pre-op room hours before the sun comes up was only slightly better than freezing to death in a meat locker. On the one hand, it was cold. On the other, it was boring. Pre-op rooms, like operating rooms, are kept unusually cool to slow the growth of bacteria that can lead to dangerous infections. And at barely 5:00 AM, there wasn't a line, or much of anything else. When your nurse finished prepping you, you were pretty much alone with your saline drip until your doctor showed up.

For Jeff that wouldn't be for a while. Dr. Maciunas was running late. Jeff didn't mind. He had waited his whole life for this day. What was another hour?

When his doctors finally arrived it took them three hours to fit him with the titanium halo they would later bolt to the table in order to hold his head motionless for surgery. They put two screws into his temple and two more near each cheek.

To Jeff the halo just seemed like a cool, high-tech face mask. "Can I have this when this is all over?" he asked.

"Sure," Maciunas said. "If you have $86,000."

After making sure the halo was secure, doctors took Jeff for a quick MRI to ensure that it was properly aligned. Then they left to prepare for the operation. There was nothing to do but wait in the cold, lonely room, so the nurses bent the rules and let Jeff's family in to help pass the time. At 9:15 AM the six family members who made it to the hospital—his mother, father, brother, Debra, Aunt Suzie, and cousin Kelly—gathered slowly around his bed.

"What's up, guys," Jeff said.

As they looked at Jeff their eyes narrowed as if to say, "What is that thing on your head?"

"Gosh, does that hurt?" Aunt Suzie asked, getting so close to his face she could see the deep indentations made by the screws. She covered her mouth with her hand and said, "I'm sorry. I didn't mean that."

"No," Jeff said. "It's totally cool."

Then she turned to her sister, Jeff's mother. "Look how deep those screws are," she said.

Jeff looked at his older brother, who had never been comfortable around blood or medical procedures. His face was turning white and he seemed a tad wobbly. Jeff reached over with his left arm and grabbed a glass of orange juice. "Steve, want some OJ?" he said. "You're looking a little pale, there."

Then he yelled to the reception nurse at the desk. "Hey, you mind if we get some chairs?" he said. "We're having a party in here. I'm about to change my life today."

She laughed and brought over chairs that they arranged in a semicircle around the bed. Some sat. Others stood. His parents sat closest to him, on his right. His father looked at his youngest son and shook his head. His mother reached out to put both of her hands on top of Jeff's right hand, which was resting on the gurney. Then his father did the same, putting both of his hands on top of her hands. Jeff looked at both of their hands touching his and smiled softly. As he looked into their eyes, all three of them welled up with tears. In the silence Jeff promised he would remember that moment forever.

"Well, Jeff," his dad said. "After this operation you might not be able to share so many of your funny stories with us anymore."

"Speaking of those stories," Jeff said. "Why don't we tell a few now?"

People with Tourette's *always* had stories. And while waiting for surgery, Jeff delivered his like a stand-up comic. He told about the time at the dentist when he ticked so hard the curved, plastic suction device flew out of his mouth and began sucking on his neck. He told about the time when a pharmacist thought he was flirting with her when he tried to hand her a twenty-dollar bill only to have an arm tic repeatedly pull it back before she could take it.

"And one day I was walking in the parking lot at Target—" Jeff said.

"Oh, you guys are gonna love this one!" Steve said, a smile of recognition crossing his face.

"And I see my friend Pete from college," Jeff said. "He's walking with his parents. I see them approaching, and I'm like, 'Oh no.' At least Pete knew about my tics. So, they come up and Pete introduces me, and his father extends his hand, you know, like, 'Nice to meet you, Jeff.' It went fine at first. I put out my hand and shook his. But then—"

"Uh-oh," someone said, sensing the story was about to take a weird turn.

"My hand contracted really hard, and I put a death grip on him, squeezing him so tightly he couldn't break free."

"Oh no!" Aunt Suzie gasped.

"Oh yeah!" Jeff said. "And then I yanked my arm—and his—back really hard," he said, clenching his right fist and pumping his arm violently back toward his body two times in a row. "He couldn't understand what I was doing. He just screamed. You know, 'Aaaah-hhh! How dare you, you freak? What are you trying to do to me?' And then his wife yelled too. 'What are you doing to my husband? Help! Helllllp!' "

His family broke out laughing. "Oh, God," Jeff said. "I told him I was so sorry. But he wasn't in any mood to listen. When he finally managed pull his hand out of my sweaty grasp, he started quickly back for the car holding his hand as if he had just been mauled by a grizzly bear. His wife ran after him. 'How's your hand? How's your hand?' " Jeff said, affecting an elderly woman's voice.

"Pete just looked at me. He was like, 'Don't worry about it. I'll explain it to them on the ride home.' "

The stories just kept coming. He told of the time he felt a massive tic coming on while riding alone in a department store elevator. When he finally expressed it—bending at the knees and clenching his fists as he screamed, red-faced, with all his strength—the doors had opened to reveal a little old woman with eyes the size of silver dollars. She dropped her purse, started screaming, threw her hands up in the air, and ran the other way.

His family couldn't catch their breath. After several more stories, they were all laughing so loudly a nurse had to tell them to pipe down because they were disturbing the other patients.

Jeff was just thankful for the laughter. He didn't want the last memory his family had of him to be that of someone who was worried or scared.

— —

AND THEN IT was time.

As Maciunas washed up, two doctors in powder-blue scrubs with white masks hanging loosely around their chins—one young, the other middle-aged—walked in the room.

"Ready to get this show on the road?" they asked.

"Today's the beginning of a new life for me," Jeff said. "Let's do this."

With Jeff sitting at a forty-five-degree angle, the doctors put the side rails of the gurney up and got on either side.

"Do you want your family to walk with you?" one asked.

"They're coming with me because they're going to live my new life with me," Jeff said.

His family walked beside him as the doctors rolled him slowly toward the operating room. With each squeak of the gurney's wheels, it became increasingly more real. This was it. This was happening. Tears began to fall. He looked into the faces of the people he loved the most in the world. They were more emotional than he had ever seen them.

They didn't know what to think. Were they wishing him good luck on a new life? Or saying good-bye to him for the last time? Jeff maintained his composure. He didn't cry. He even managed a smile and an "I love you" as he gave each one a kiss.

"I'll see you on the flip side," he said. "And you can quote me on that."

He turned and flashed one last smile as the doors to the operating room closed and locked with a loud click. For Jeff it was a powerful moment. The doors symbolized the end of one chapter of his life and the beginning of another. This was the new frontier. *This* was hope.

Jeff looked back through the small windows in the doors and whispered to himself.

"My past is out there," he said. "My future's in here."

AS A SMALL group of doctors and nurses swirled around him, Jeff couldn't help but wonder if all was all going as planned. He wanted to ask but didn't dare interrupt them, especially during their most delicate work.

He needn't have worried. The operation, which lasted roughly eight hours and ended at 4:00 PM, went as well as his doctors could have hoped. Working slowly and carefully, they followed a meticulous plan and detailed computer models to successfully implant the tiny electrodes, called stimulators, deep in his brain.

There was no infection. No excessive bleeding. And while they still couldn't be sure it ultimately would work, all indications were that they had hit their target. It wouldn't be long before they would know for sure.

Eleven days later, Jeff would undergo a second surgery to have two rectangular battery packs implanted in his pectoral muscles. The plan was to use those battery packs, connected by fine wires to the stimulators, to send electrical pulses into Jeff's brain in an attempt to interrupt and correct the misfiring signals thought to be causing his tics.

After the operation, nurses removed the halo around Jeff's head and wheeled him into a recovery room in the intensive care unit. As he struggled to open his eyes in the dimly lit room he saw members of his family coming in. Drugs kept him relaxed, while the swelling in his brain worked to reduce his tics.

He looked at Debra with searching eyes and spoke in a groggy voice. "Did it go OK?" he said.

With tears welling up, Debra looked at her husband and bent down to kiss him on his cheek. She took his hand.

"Yes, honey," she said. "The doctors said it went well."

Later Jeff asked his doctors the same question and got the same answer.

Still, he kept asking. "You're *sure* it went OK?" he asked Debra again.

"Yes, dear," she said. Debra wanted to project a confident and strong front. But inside she was scared. Sure, *this* operation had worked. But what about the next one? And then what? Would they work like they all hoped? Would Jeff be able to be the husband and father he longed to be? Or would he go back to being bedridden again? She swallowed hard. There were no guarantees.

But as concerned as Debra was, it was Jeff's father who felt the worst after the operation. "Did it work?" he asked the doctors following the operation. "Is . . . is he better?"

"We won't know that until after the next operation and we can see if everything works the way we hope it will," Dr. Maciunas said.

Jim Matovic's head dropped. *Next* surgery? Jeff had not told his father much about deep brain stimulation. He had not told him it wouldn't work right away. He had not told him it had two parts. And he certainly hadn't told him that it had never before worked on someone with Tourette Syndrome. After the disappointing news, Jeff's father had to walk off by himself to be alone with his emotions.

Jeff spent thirty-six hours in the ICU before being transferred to a regular room. As time crawled, his mind raced. Monitors hummed as he stared at the ceiling and thought about his future. He could hardly believe it. This was really happening—and he had already made it past the hardest part!

He thought about his next surgery and the exciting times ahead.

"Just a matter of time now, he thought. "Just a matter of time."

42

Turn Me On, Tina

TWO WEEKS AFTER doctors implanted battery packs in his chest walls, Jeff was ready for the biggest test of all.

March 4, 2004. For weeks he had stared at the date on his calendar. It was either going to be the best day of his life or the worst. That was the day he would find out if the operation worked, the day he would find out if he had a future, the day they *finally* would switch on his stimulators.

That morning Jeff pulled on gray shorts and a white T-shirt, and his father drove him to the hospital. They parked on the fourth floor of the parking garage and then took the elevator down. As they walked up the steps to University Hospitals, Jeff's body went into a spasm, moving him up and down, up and down. Jim Matovic reached out to help his son, to no avail. It was like holding hands with a yo-yo. Jeff grunted, forcefully expelled air from his mouth, then unleashed violent clenched-fist punches into the air that could have could have put a heavyweight boxer on his butt. Jeff walked like a drunken sailor with exaggerated, pounding steps. Sometimes they looked purposeful and angry, as if he were on a mission to do harm. Other times it looked more like he was trying to stamp out a cigarette butt. As he walked, his eyes twitched, his head rolled, and his neck snapped.

Once inside, he and his father were quickly ushered into a small room in the neurology department on the hospital's sixth floor. They were joined by neurologist Brian Maddux, Jim Adler of Medtronic, and clinical nurse specialist Tina Whitney.

Jeff sat in a chair as best he could. A small crowd gathered around—Maddux to his right, Whitney and Adler to his left, and his father directly in front of him.

"Are we ready to begin?" asked Whitney, a small, blonde-haired specialist who took the lead role in adjusting Jeff's stimulators.

Jeff nodded yes, and everyone seemed to lean in just a little closer.

Armed with a stylus and a black device slightly larger than a smartphone, Whitney activated the stimulators and began the slow and artful process of tuning him in like a radio. She used her handheld computer to communicate, one by one, with two pulse generators implanted just under Jeff's collarbone. The computer communicated by telemetry through Jeff's clothes and his skin. Each electrode in Jeff's brain had four leads. Tuning the orchestra in his head, as his doctors often put it, would be neither easy nor quick.

Maddux didn't know what to expect. He didn't know if the stimulation would have an immediate effect, a delayed effect, or no effect. Whitney adjusted the amplitude (the strength) and the rate (the frequency) of the pulses-per-second stimulation, which could go as high as 185 pulses per second. She also adjusted the length of each pulse, measured in microseconds. Over several hours she patiently tried countless combinations. Able to work on one side of his body at a time, she tried low frequencies and high frequencies, narrow pulse widths and wide pulse widths. One adjustment made Jeff's vision blurry. Another made him dizzy. After a third, he couldn't swallow correctly. But after almost an hour of adjustments, his tics hadn't improved.

Although Jeff had been told the process could take some time, his head dropped. He couldn't help but worry that the operation had failed. *Oh well*, he thought. *At least I tried. And that was worth something.*

But just as he convinced himself nothing was going to happen, it did. The feeling was subtle at first, but it was something. He had never felt anything like this before. It was indescribable—a calmness, a relaxation of tension, a modicum of control. Was he imagining it? No! Whitney's adjustments had made a difference. Suddenly Jeff's tics began to lessen. Whitney noticed. So did Jeff.

"Is that better?" she said.

"Absolutely!" a stunned Jeff said.

And then, with a few more adjustments, Whitney hit frequency-modulation gold! Within thirty seconds the four leads on one of the electrodes in Jeff's brain began producing a series of pulses that caused his tics to virtually disappear on the left side of his body. He stopped twitching. He stopped punching. He stopped jerking and kicking and clearing his throat. More important, the urges that drove those movements disappeared as well.

Jeff said nothing, almost unable to process what was happening in his body. As wonderful as it was to have the tics gone on his left side, he had now become a strange creature, with powerful movements still ruling his right side.

His father shook his head as tears rolled down his cheek. He couldn't believe his eyes. Half of his son was calm, relaxed, silent. "It's like you glued two different bodies together, but kept the clothing the same," he said.

Just then Whitney spoke. "Sorry, but I have to try another combo," she said.

A singular thought ran through Jim Matovic's mind: *Are you crazy? Leave it here! It works!*

At the same time Jeff had a fearful thought. What if Whitney couldn't repeat the success on the right side? But she wasn't about to let that happen.

Two hours passed.

Nothing. Jeff kept ticking and kicking . . . until . . .

Whitney noticed a change in Jeff's motions.

"Did you feel something there?" she said.

"I think so," Jeff said. "Yeah. I think so."

After a few more adjustments, the tics on Jeff's right side noticeably decreased. Then she added the settings for the left. In thirty seconds the last of his tics—on both sides—simply and quietly melted away. His arms and legs fell quiet. No one talked. In the silence of the room Jeff's body became perfectly still. Mouths hung open. Against all odds it had worked. For the first time in history, deep brain stimulation had completely worked on someone with Tourette Syndrome!

Jeff looked stunned as his new, calm body actually responded to his control. He breathed as if taking a breath for the first time. His muscles relaxed and his eyes fluttered as if he were waking up in a whole new world. Maddux looked at Whitney in shock. There were no words. Out of nowhere, Geppetto's puppet had come to life!

Jeff's father bent in front of his son like a catcher in a crouch, mouth open, eyes wide with wonder. His son was back! After thirty years it was more than he could take. Weeping openly, he couldn't have imagined a greater miracle.

Neither could Jeff. "I . . . I've never experienced this before," he said.

Jeff tried to talk further but stumbled over his words. His eyes darted left, then right, looking at nothing. With all his attention focused inward, he kept waiting for a tic, a twitch, a jerk, a spasm. He kept waiting for his tics to come back, for his speech to be interrupted.

It felt wonderful but foreign. All the sensations he had grown used to disappeared in an instant. It was strange looking at his father. Rather, it was strange looking at him straight on, without having to correct for blinking eyes or a violently jerking head.

He was not used to this. This was *not* him. But it felt unbelievable!

Jeff hugged his father, then began to cry. An odd sense of peace washed over every muscle in his body. And he could talk—fluidly, without interruption. It was impossible, like some sort of dream, but it was true. He was *normal* again.

A shocked Brian Maddux called his partner, neurosurgeon Robert Maciunas. "You've got to come and see this!" he said.

After a few more moments, it was time to take Jeff 2.0 for a test drive. Sure, Jeff felt better while he was seated. But how would he do when he was really moving? He walked several steps around the office. His muscles felt smooth and under control. Whitney shone a laser pointer on the wall.

"See the red dot?" she said. "Point at it."

Boom! No hesitation. Jeff put his finger dead on it.

"Jeff, now I'd like you to walk down the hallway," Maddux said. And just like that, Jeff did. He walked, calmly, leisurely, down the hallway. He smiled as he stopped to look at and read everything on the wall. No punches. No kicks.

Jim Matovic just shook his head, and looked at Dr. Maddux as if to ask, *Do you see what I see? And do you believe what you're seeing?*

Thank you, God! Jim Matovic thought.

Jeff couldn't believe his sudden stillness either. He picked up a magazine.

"Dad, I can *read* this!" he said.

"I know! I know!" his crying father said.

"Look! I can hold a cup!"

For several minutes he kept stating random things he could do to anyone who would listen.

Back in the hall he made eye contact with a nurse who was passing by. "Hey!" he said in an uncomfortably loud and cheerful voice. "How are you today?"

"Umm, OK." the nurse said. "How are you?"

"FANTASTIC!" Jeff said.

He continued walking around the hallway, interacting with anybody or anything, doing things he never thought he'd ever be able to do again. An ocean of stillness took over his body.

Suddenly everything was amazing. He stood up. *Standing was amazing!* He sat back down. *Sitting was even better!* After a few more minutes, Maciunas walked in the room and looked at the man he had healed.

There'd be time for thank-yous later. Right then, Jeff was too busy pointing out things he could do. "Dad, Dad," he said, putting his finger on a hospital evacuation plan on the wall. "If there's a fire, this is where we need to go! And *this* is where we are!"

"That's great, Jeff!" his father said.

"Want me to turn the lights on?" he said. "Off? On? 'Cause I can do it!"

He stood on his right leg and held out his arms while lifting his left leg in front of him at a forty-five-degree angle. "Dad, check this out," he said.

Jeff then glanced at Maciunas and Maddux and flashed them a smile. He had never seen two doctors more speechless in his life. He kept waiting for a tic or a twitch. It never came.

He was normal. *Normal!* It was everything he had been praying for. After handshakes, hugs, and tearful thank-yous, Jeff walked back to the car beside his father without a single tic. No movements! No sounds! No grunting! No fist punching!

When they reached the elevator in the parking garage, they stopped. Then, in the echoing silence, they turned and looked at each other with a similar thought. "Let's take the stairs!" they said together, suddenly realizing that Jeff could. Such a little thing. But it was *everything*.

From that day forward, Jim Matovic would always think of March 4 as the day his son "marched forth" into a new life.

43

"Welcome Back to Your Life"

THEY COULDN'T WAIT to share the news. Jeff had been healed! Not just helped, *healed*! As in no more grunting, no more punching, no more head shaking or eye blinking. No more tics of any kind!

Doctors were careful not to use the word *cured*. The tics were still there, they said. They were just being controlled by the stimulators.

Who cares? Jeff thought. For him it was the same thing. For the first time in more than three decades he could relax!

As Jim Matovic drove his son home he called his wife, Patty, on his cell phone. But when she answered, he couldn't speak.

"Hello?" Patty Matovic said. "Hello?"

Jim handed the phone to Jeff, who told his mother the news. "Mom," he said. "It worked."

He heard screams through the phone. "Oh, Jeffrey," she said. "That's *wonderful* news! I just can't believe it! It worked?"

"It worked, Mom. All my tics are gone!"

Her prayers had been answered. Her son was all better. No more tics! No more pain or suffering! But it still seemed so unreal. She couldn't wait to see him for herself.

A few minutes later, Jeff's father called Debra. She had been waiting all day for news, had even eaten lunch at her desk. If she hadn't exhausted all of her vacation days, she would have been there with Jeff herself. But she didn't dare ask for another day or risk getting caught calling in sick. Besides, doctors had cautioned them that they would likely have to come back several times for numerous adjustments and not to expect anything to happen at the first appointment.

Debra grabbed the phone on its first ring, only to hear her father-in-law sobbing on the other end. For a moment her entire world went dark. *Oh God*, she thought, *it hasn't gone well!*

But then—what was that?—she heard laughing over the crying. "What's going on here?" she said. "Dad. Tell me. What's happened?"

"Deb," Jeff's father said. "Deb, it worked!"

"Huh?" Debra said, perking up. "How much? Tell me what percentage we're at here. What's still going?"

"I'm going to put Jeff on. He'll tell you."

"HONEY!" Jeff shouted excitedly into the phone. "I have no tics! I haven't ticked *once* since whatever time we started!"

"Are you *joking*?" Debra said, excited, but aware that Jeff was famous for his practical jokes. "You're not pulling my leg here?"

"No, I'm not," Jeff said. "You know I wouldn't joke about this!" Deb's mouth hung open. Best-case scenario, she had thought, maybe—if they were lucky—he'd see a 50 percent reduction. And now he was telling her it was 100 percent? No more tics? Not one? It was literally the best moment in her life.

She stood up and screamed into the phone. "Oh my God!" she hollered. "Oh my God! It worked! It worked!" Her coworkers began streaming out of their offices. Debra was nearly hyperventilating.

It was everything Debra could have wanted. She couldn't believe it. "It worked?" she asked again.

"It worked," Jeff said. "And it's fantastic!"

"Oh, I love you so much!" she said. "I'm so happy for you, and I can't wait to see you!"

They spoke for several minutes before Jeff had to end the call.

"We're going to go get some lunch now," he said. "We haven't had anything to eat."

"OK," Debra said, still vibrating with excitement. "OK, you go do that, and I'll see you at home."

She couldn't wait till the end of the day.

Jeff and his father, still reeling from the events at the hospital, stopped to pick up some hamburgers from Burger King, then continued their drive to Jeff's house. They drove in silence. No music. Not even much talking. Jeff was having too much fun looking out the window, looking at houses and trees, and trying to orient himself to this new world he was seeing. Nothing was shaking. His world was unusually still. He reached out with a steady hand and felt the air. *This is wonderful,* he thought.

Jim Matovic thought the same thing. But he couldn't help but be wary. As he drove, he glanced at his son every several seconds to check for a shake, a twitch, *something.*

There was nothing. He wanted to be giddy. But questions gnawed at him. Would Jeff's stillness last an hour? A week? Or was it—he almost didn't want to say it out loud for fear of jinxing it—*permanent?*

No one knew, not even his doctors.

When they arrived back at Jeff's house, they made one more call— to Jeff's brother. Steve, an engineer, worked as a manager at a gear manufacturing company. He took the call in his office.

"Uh, Steve," Jeff said laughing and yelling into the phone at the same time. "It worked! It worked!"

"What's that?" Steve said, trying to hear over the noise. He shut his office door. "What? What's going on? Where are you right now?"

"I'm at my place, and I'm not ticking," Jeff said. "I haven't ticked for hours."

"Your whole body?" Steve said.

"Yeah!"

Jeff heard Steve call to his boss in a loud voice. "Jim," he said, "I'm going to be gone the rest of the day." Then he addressed Jeff again. "I'll be over in a minute," he said. "This is wonderful! I can't wait to see you."

When Steve arrived at Jeff's house, he hesitated for a moment when he saw Jeff standing still beside their father in the dining room. He walked quickly across the floor toward him, walking faster the closer he got. With tears streaming down his face, he grabbed Jeff and held him in a tight embrace. He didn't let go for several minutes. He just rocked back and forth, patting him on the back. Jeff started to cry.

"Welcome back, Jeff," Steve said. "Welcome back to your life!"

One by one the people in Jeff's life began showing up for the celebration. As friends and family looked at him, they held their breath. It was as if he were fragile, and they didn't want to be the one to "break" him.

Deb got to go home an hour and a half after getting the news. She drove home as fast as she could. When she finally walked in the door, she saw Jeff's father and brother, both with huge grins on their faces. Then she looked at Jeff, and he looked back at her. It was incredible! Finally, the man she had always seen on the inside was standing there the way she had always pictured him in her mind. The gleam in his eyes, the smile on his face. And it wasn't just her who could see it anymore. It was everyone. *Everyone* could see it!

They didn't say a word as, for a moment, the world stood still. Crying, she walked up to him and got lost in his huge embrace.

Later that night, after the celebrating was over and everyone had gone home, Jeff enjoyed his newfound stillness on the basketball court in his driveway. It was so amazing just to be able to hold the ball without ticking. In the dim of the evening he stood at the free-throw line for the longest time just bouncing the ball. He stood there, alone in the driveway, for ten minutes without taking a single shot.

"Well look at me," he said to himself. "I'm holding the ball."

The little things were everything. Holding a ball. Grabbing a tissue and blowing his nose. Getting an actual glass out of the cupboard instead of a sippy cup! Every experience, no matter how small, was a brand-new miracle.

Days went by. Then weeks. No tics. Not one.

Aunt Suzie, Jeff's cousin Kelly, and his grandmother came to visit.

"Just look at him!" Deb said, showing Jeff off like a new car.

Finally, after weeks went by with no regression, they decided to celebrate. They took the kids and went to Applebee's for dinner.

For the first time since she had met him, Debra was able to go to a restaurant with Jeff without having anyone stare or point. She watched in amazement as he cut up his steak without silverware flying everywhere! He had never been more proud. Suddenly he wanted to do everything!

"Let's go to the mall!" Jeff said. "Let's go to the movies! I want to see the most action-packed movie you can find!"

Days later he returned to St. Francis Chapel. The building was empty. His eyes never left the crucifix as he prayed out loud. "I can't thank you enough, God," he said. "My life has changed because of the blessings that you have provided me in terms of the people, the support, and the technology—down to the last janitor at Medtronic."

He thanked God for a multitude of new blessings and for his new life. He knelt before the altar and bent down low as he gently kissed the top step. Before he left, he stopped to turn back the pages in the prayer book to the original prayer he had written in it. It read: "God, please let this surgery work."

Jeff's lip trembled as he put a check mark by it. Then he took a pen and wrote one more note in the book. It read, simply, "Thanks so much."

44

Telling the World

IF JEFF DIDN'T know what a media circus was before the operation, it didn't take long for him to find out. About a month after doctors turned on his stimulators, University Hospitals held a news conference to tell the world. Several dozen reporters and cameramen gathered at the hospital.

An administrator showed a video of Jeff's journey. Then she introduced the guests of honor.

Dr. Robert Maciunas spoke first. "What's especially thrilling to us at the University Hospitals of Cleveland and our Movement Disorders Center is that, in this case, Jeff Matovic's leap of faith has the potential for becoming a great step forward for selected patients with Tourette Syndrome," he said. "In February he underwent that surgery—went through it successfully—and this little pacemaker was then activated in March with the results that you've seen both on the videotape and by Jeffrey Matovic walking in here and sitting calmly in that chair."

Later in the news conference, he praised Jeff's courage. "It's one thing for me, as a surgeon with experience in deep brain stimulator surgery . . . to feel confident that something makes sense neurologically, and that something could be predicted to work," he said. "It's quite another . . . for a young man to lie down upon an operating table and say 'Let's do this' with all the hope in the world. I couldn't have expected more from a patient like Jeff. . . . We're thrilled! . . . Jeff has had a spectacular result."

Dr. David Riley, chair of the hospital's Movement Disorders Center, then told the crowd what Jeff's operation meant to him. "I have the excitement of knowing that I have another tool . . . to work against this disorder [with] people who do have severe enough symptoms to be treated [with DBS]."

During her talk, Dr. Tina Whitney described the excitement of turning on Jeff's stimulators. "As I am adjusting the stimulator, I am observing Jeff," she said. "I am looking to see if his tics are decreasing in frequency or intensity, or if he is experiencing any adverse effects from the stimulation. After about two hours of adjusting the stimulator. . . . Wow! I don't know what else to say but wow! The outcome of that day was beyond *any* of our expectations. For the first time in years Jeff was sitting still. He was able to drink from a glass of water without spilling. He could hold a piece of paper and read it without losing his place. He was able to walk normally, and he was sitting calmly. I look at Jeff, and he's got a grin from ear to ear. I look at dad. Dad's tearful. I'm tearful. I mean, it was really an incredibly emotional day for all of us. . . . I want to thank Jeff for his courage, and for putting his trust in us."

Then it was Jeff's turn. He walked calmly and confidently to the podium as the clicking of dozens of camera shutters echoed through the room.

"Good morning, everyone," he said. "First of all I want to send a great, huge thank-you to my family: my wife, Debra; my kids, who are not here; and my parents, Jim and Patty Matovic; my brother, Steve; his wife, Lisa. It's been a long, long time. But this is truly the day of my life in terms of where I hoped to go for so long. So for all those doctor's appointments, visits, and whatnot, I can't say enough thanks. A special thanks to University Hospital's surgical team, especially Dr. Maciunas and Dr. Maddux, Dr. Whitney, and all the people who helped out to make this such a successful thing.

"I remember [as] a child being very different. . . . So many people in this world strive to be extraordinary. What I wanted to do was be like everybody else."

He talked about what he treasured most in his new life. "The simple things in life that I took for granted," he said. "I can pick up this glass of water and hold it and drink it. I can walk with it, and do so many things that before were just figments of my imagination. . . . And managing my own goals and strengths without the need for wondering what the outcome will be. . . . I certainly want to be a friend and an advocate for anyone out there, any families that are struggling, looking for some sign of hope, some sign of courage, and the opportunity to find strength."

His family spoke next, starting with his mother. "Well, what a day!" a smiling Patty Matovic said. She talked briefly about Jeff's childhood, then addressed his struggles as he grew up. "It was a difficult time for him in that there were moments when I am sure that he lost hope," she said. "And what I'd like to say is to tell Jeff how proud of him his family is. We watched it happen. He lived it. We could tell that there were times when Jeff thought, *What is living all about? Maybe it would be easier if I weren't.* Those were very dark days. The strength that Jeff displayed during this time allowed him to make many friends, it allowed him to excel in sports, it allowed him to graduate from college. It was this same strength in his faith in God that allowed him to go to that operating room. He *fought* for February 9, 2004. . . . And Jeff is truly our hero."

Jeff's father then had his turn. "I think Tina said it best," he said. "Just wow! I was there when Jeff got turned on. And when chins dropped down to about here—enough said. I guess I get to say some thanks too. But how does one really say thank you for a miracle? I can think of my dad, and he would just tell me, 'Keep it simple and say it from the heart.' But thank you just doesn't seem adequate. *Thank you.* They're simple words. Know that they come from the deepest part of our hearts."

He thanked God "who orchestrated this entire journey," his family and friends "who were there during the hard times to give us a shoulder to lean on, or to cry on," and the people in prayer groups whose prayers "were heard loud and clear."

"And the surgical team," he said. "Dr. Maciunas and his group. What can we say to them? Yes, it was a chance, and it was risky on both sides. But, I think, there's only one word that comes to my head when I look at and think about the results that they produced, and it's one of Jeff's favorite words: *awesome*! That fits, and I think that's the only one that really does fit. Something that will always remain with me as an indelible memory occurred when our son, Steve, saw Jeff for the first time after the batteries were turned on and very simply told him 'Welcome back, Jeff. Welcome back.'"

Steve stepped to the microphone. *"Welcome back* was probably the right thing to say because he was a whole new person," he said. "I'd say for the last ten years I haven't seen Jeff the way I saw him when he got back from the doctor's office. And it *was* awesome. . . . The reason, I think, that Jeff's favorite word is *awesome* is because he truly is. There's a strength that I never knew he had. And it took that kind of strength to get through everything that he got through over the past ten years. He's taught me a lot about what it means to be strong. He's taught our family what it means to be faithful. And I think he's going to be a wonderful example for other people who suffer from Tourette's. There's not much else to say. It's just wonderful to have him back."

Then Debra joined Jeff at the podium for questions. A female reporter asked him how his new life felt. "I'm still getting used to walking around the house and instead of getting the plastic cup with the sipper lid, I am able to grab a glass. I am able to . . . groom myself, and those sorts of things."

"What's it been like for Bonnie and Michael?"

"The one thing that they've commented on is 'Gee, Dad's pretty still,'" Jeff said. "The other thing is they kind of miss me bumping 'em when I am ticking, or throwing things around. They think that's kind of neat. But . . . they have certainly been very, very responsive and very happy and encouraging."

"Can you describe what your first steps were like?"

"I don't think I can even use my own word—*awesome*—to describe what that was like. I think the best analogy was when Tina turned the left side of my body on, which is the right stimulator in my brain, I was walking down the hallway as Dr. Maddux was there and Tina, and [my left side] is just walking smoothly, calm as anything, and this side's still ticking. So, it was basically like you had two different vertical people put together, which was pretty interesting. In terms of what I feel now, I'm getting used to it. I'm enjoying it, and certainly going from there."

"Is there anything you can't do because you have electrodes in your head? Can you . . . not go through metal detectors?"

"I have to be a little more careful at the airports," Jeff said. "Fortunately I have cards that I carry with me that I can display to anyone who would want to run a scan over my body. The other thing I have been provided with is my own remote control, if you will. It's about the size of a small television remote control. I have the ability to turn my batteries on and off. I usually don't touch those buttons—*unless* I go to a store and their theft deterrent system turns my batteries off . . . I can reactivate them."

"Jeff, what made you want to be the first [DBS patient] *in North America, knowing all the risks and possible downsides and unknowns of having the surgery?"*

"Actually I didn't know that I was [the first] until afterward," Jeff said. "But I was really pinned in a corner. . . . I think it's a lot of faith in God, and faith and belief and an attitude that I'm going to get through this. . . . I certainly hope to have conveyed that message to other people who could benefit from the surgery."

After more than an hour, the news conference concluded with a question for Debra.

"You must have met him when he was—"

"Still ticking, yeah," Debra said.

"What did you see in him? I mean, he couldn't have been the smoothest Casanova."

"It's a funny thing about Tourette's and patients who suffer from this," Debra said. "On some subconscious level, when they meet someone for the very first time, they are actually able to suppress their tics. . . . So the first thing I saw from him were some great big brown eyes, a big ol' smile on his face, and him saying, 'Hey, those are really nice boots!' But what did I see in him?" Debra asked herself, gazing at her husband. "I just saw everything."

45

Oprah and Good Morning America

IT DIDN'T TAKE long for the news to spread.

"Excuse me," a hospital representative said after the news conference, extending her cell phone toward Jeff. "I have Thea Trachtenburg from ABC on the phone. Can you take the call?"

ABC? Jeff thought. *What do* they *want?* They wanted an interview. Live in New York—on *Good Morning America.*

Jeff had barely finished a news conference in Cleveland. How did they know already in New York? But after more calls from around the country—and around the world—it dawned on him. He had ceased to be Jeff Matovic of Cleveland, Ohio, and had become "Jeff Matovic, international news story."

By the weekend, Jeff and Debra had flown to New York to do *Good Morning America.* As they waited in the greenroom, coanchor Diane Sawyer—who had been previewing the story all morning—stopped in to wish Jeff and Debra good luck. Later, after getting their makeup done, they listened as Sawyer introduced them.

"The next story is about a young man, and we've been talking about it all morning, and all during the break, and you're just not going to believe it," she said.

On set with Sawyer, Charlie Gibson, and ABC's medical editor Dr. Tim Johnson, Jeff and Debra stared into a bank of white-hot lights and tried to calm their racing hearts. It was their first time on national television, and it wasn't at all what they envisioned. The same set that looked huge at home wasn't that big in person—not that much larger than a typical living room. What was different was the nonstop activity. Stagehands scuttled around, directors barked instructions, and wires curled across the floor like dozens of long, black snakes. Debra shifted in her seat and managed a smile as she took a deep breath as if to say *We can do this.*

Large cameras pointed at them, ready to beam their story to the world. It was time.

Gibson, the veteran news anchor, took his seat facing them. He smiled warmly, then extended his hand. "Hey," he said with a calming voice of an old pro. "Relex. Just be yourselves with this."

Out of the corner of her eye Debra could see Sawyer sitting at the anchor desk about one hundred feet away in front of a live audience. Behind Gibson, Jeff could see Matthew Perry of *Friends* sitting in a leather recliner getting ready for his interview.

When the cameras rolled, Jeff recounted his remarkable story from beginning to end. Even he didn't quite believe it as the words came out of his mouth about Tourette's, deep brain stimulation, and his miracle. As he told the story Gibson just shook his head as if to say "Wow!"

Bonnie and Mike watched the interview from the side. At one point Gibson asked Debra what made her fall in love with Jeff. She looked at her husband, then back at Gibson.

"That smile," she said, flashing one of her own. "Who wouldn't love that?"

Before they knew it, they were done. The anchors shook their heads in amazement and cut to a commercial. Afterward the anchors told the couple how blown away they were by the story's emotional power and how honored they were to have delivered Jeff's message of hope.

"This has to be one of the top five stories we've ever covered in terms of a pure, groundbreaking, feel-good story," Sawyer said.

Jeff couldn't believe that. *These people have interviewed presidents and celebrities. And for her to say that ...*

Matthew Perry had watched them in amazement. Jeff recognized him immediately as he walked toward him across the set.

"Mr. Perry, it's a pleasure to meet you," he said. Perry looked up and cocked his head.

"Now how in the hell am I supposed to top that?" he said, pretending to get up and walk out. "I'm leaving!" Sawyer, Gibson, and the film crew burst out laughing.

Perry then got serious. "In all honesty, what you've done—taking that chance and putting your life on the line for others—that's bigger news that I'll ever make," Perry said. "You've just shocked the world! I hope your lives turn out to be everything you want, because of anyone I've ever met who deserves it, it's you."

"Thank you," Jeff said, searching for something to say in return. "And I just want you to know I'm a huge fan."

"Well, I've just become one of your number-one fans too," Perry said with a smile. "With that, my friend. I salute you."

A WEEK AFTER appearing on *Good Morning America*, Jeff got a call from Molly O'Connor, a producer for an even bigger program. "I'm calling from *The Oprah Winfrey Show*," she said. "Oprah asked me to give you a call."

Jeff's heart jumped into his throat. "Is this a joke?" he asked.

"No joke," O'Connor said.

For a moment Jeff couldn't speak.

"Jeff?"

"That would be awesome!" Jeff said.

"Great. We just heard about your miraculous surgery, and Oprah would be honored to have you on her show."

"Yeah. That's amazing. Thank you. But . . . could I ask you something?"

"Anything," O'Connor said.

"It would mean the world to me to have my parents out there with me. Is there any way they could be brought out for the show too?"

"Absolutely," O'Connor said.

Later, Jeff called his mother. "How'd you like to come out to the *Oprah* show with us?"

"We're already coming!" his mother said. "Molly just called us!"

Days later they all landed in Chicago. The show put them up in the Omni Hotel, a towering, all-suite property on North Michigan Avenue.

The next day a black stretch limousine with a wet bar, stereo, and a TV took them to the taping. When they pulled up to the studio, two enormous security guards—both at least six foot seven with three hundred pounds of bulging muscle stuffed into black T-shirts with Harpo logos—walked them inside the door. At only 185 pounds, Jeff felt as if they could have eaten him for breakfast.

Security at the *Oprah* show was tighter than at any airport. Guards took cell phones and cameras and then started scanning everyone with handheld metal detectors. The largest guard, with biceps so huge they prevented his arms from hanging straight down from his body, took a step toward Jeff.

Jeff and Debra both threw their hands up and said, "You can't do that."

"It's policy," he said with a voice worthy of James Earl Jones. "I'm sorry."

"You *can't* do that," Jeff repeated, stepping back. "You don't understand. I have batteries. You'll turn them off!"

"I *have to,*" the guard said.

"You do it and you might as well call 9-1-1 right now," Debra said. "Because you will not have a show."

"Well, you might have a show, but it won't be any kind of show you'll want to see," Jeff said. Sure, Jeff could use his remote to reset his device—but it took twenty seconds for the batteries to turn on. Twenty seconds of ticking would have taken a horrible toll.

Just then Molly O'Connor, the tan and pretty producer in her late twenties who invited them on the show, came running into the hallway. "Don't wand him!" she said. "It will turn off his batteries, and his Tourette's tics will come back!"

The guards looked at her.

"It's OK," she said. "Let them through."

"OK," the guard said. "You're good to go. Have a good time."

O'Connor smiled and escorted them to a waiting area.

"Whoa," Jeff said as he walked in.

The carpet in Oprah's greenroom was such a rich, pure green you could almost could taste the money. The lush, paneled room had a long wooden conference table with a high-gloss finish and nearly enough leather chairs to seat the entire roster of a Major League Baseball team. Vases of fresh-cut flowers sat on tables next to a gigantic spread of the finest fruits, meats, cheeses, vegetables, and breads. Milk and dark chocolates nestled next to red, ripe strawberries. The sterling silver ser-vice that held the coffee didn't look so much like a pot as a trophy you'd win at Wimbledon.

"Just help yourself," said O'Connor. "There's always more. And if it's not what you want, we'll get it for you."

It was there, inside Harpo Studios in Chicago, that Oprah's team gave Jeff, Debra, and Jim and Patty Matovic a verbal run-through of how the show would work.

"Her theme will play, she'll come out from her doors, and go sit down and address the audience and have a little chitchat. Then she will show a little intro video that will prep the audience in terms of what kind of hell it was you were going through. That's when she's going to bring you out through those same doors. She'll say, 'Please welcome Jeff Matovic . . .' That's when Jeff walks out and the crowd goes crazy. But just relax for now. I'll come get you when it's time."

After she left the room, Jeff looked at his father and raised his eye-brows. As he took a bite of a fancy piece of chocolate, he felt like royalty. "We could live in here and feast like kings for two weeks and still not be done," he said.

Jeff's wife and mother would have indulged as well, but before they could an attractive blonde makeup artist came in and made them up for the show. "This is special makeup and lipstick," the woman said. "Don't eat anything. We don't want you to mess up your makeup."

"Don't eat anything?" Debra said. "How is that fair?" Jeff took a bite of a strawberry the size of a small softball and winked at his wife.

After the intro, Jeff got butterflies in his stomach when an assistant with an earpiece guided him to the double-doored main entrance.

This is where the most powerful woman in the world walks through, Jeff thought. *And now I'm standing here in the same spot!*

The guy with the earpiece talked fast. "You're going to go out, walk real casual, take your time, she will extend her hand, shake her hand."

Shake her hand? Jeff thought. *No way. I'm freaking hugging Oprah!*

Then, leaning out to watch for Oprah with his finger to his ear-piece, the man brushed the lapels of Jeff's suit and checked his tie like a father would for his son. "OK," he said. "You're going to go on in five seconds. Four, three, two . . ."

As soon as Jeff took his first steps outside of the door, the crowd erupted.

In introducing Jeff, Oprah screamed, "MIRACLE MAN!" three times above the din.

Instead of walking across the stage, Jeff strode toward Debra and his parents, who were sitting in the front row. One by one he gave them hugs and kisses before returning to the stage. A beaming Winfrey extended her hand. But true to his word, Jeff leaned in and gave her a hug instead.

If it was possible, the wildly clapping audience cheered even louder. As the applause washed over him, all he could think was, *I just hugged one of the most powerful women in the world!*

After the hug, he turned to wave to the audience and it finally hit him in a way that it never had before—the operation had not only been a complete success, but it also was a very big deal. Jeff's parents thought the same thing. A chill ran through them as they heard the cheers and realized that their son's life story would be seen by viewers around the world.

The interview was wonderful. His parents even got to speak to Oprah, as did Jeff's best friend, Jay Blair, who flew in as a special guest. It had been one of the best days of their lives.

For Jeff, appearing on *Oprah* and *Good Morning America* were big honors. But two years later I helped him win an award that—to him—was even bigger.

46

Shining Star

IT WAS A simple question: "Do you think Jeff would be a good candidate for the next Shining Star of Perseverance award?" my friend John Martellaro asked me in the spring of 2006.

I slapped my forehead. "Of course!" I said. "He'd be the *perfect* candidate! I hereby nominate him!"

But let's back up.

The Shining Star of Perseverance is a national award given by the WillReturn Council of Assurant Employee Benefits, a Fortune 500 insurance company in Kansas City. The award recognizes inspiring individuals and groups who overcome disabilities to succeed in society. In the previous three years the award had been won by former Kansas senator and presidential candidate Bob Dole, outdoorsman and author Aron Ralston, and the pilot of Air Force Two, Lt. Col. Andrew Lourake.

I learned about the award in 2005 from John, who had been a reporter and restaurant critic at the *Star*. Five years earlier he left the paper for a better opportunity at a Kansas City public relations and marketing firm. Assurant, one of its clients, had just selected its 2005 recipient, Lt. Col. Lourake, the first American military pilot to return to the cockpit after an above-the-knee amputation.

John called to pitch the story. He didn't need to ask twice. I found Lt. Col. Lourake, who flew the vice president and First Lady around the world—fascinating. The next year, John visited the paper and stopped by my desk. He had heard all the amazing stories I had told him about Jeff. When he asked me if Jeff would be a good candidate for the 2006 award, I couldn't believe I hadn't thought of it myself.

"He'd be perfect!" I said. "Are you kidding me? Just give it to him right now."

With my help, John submitted Jeff's story. Later, he called back with the news. Assurant had selected Jeff as the winner of the 2006 Shining Star of Perseverance award.

I called Jeff immediately. He took the call in his three-seasons room, a glass addition to their house that he used as an office.

"Hello?" he said, reclining and putting his foot on his desk.

"Hey, partner," I said. "It's Jim."

"Hey!" he said. "How you doin'?"

"I'm hanging in there. Listen, I just wanted to tell you that last year I wrote a story about a guy who won this national award called the Shining Star of Perseverance. They bring the winner to Kansas City, put 'em up in a great hotel, pay for a fancy dinner, and give them the award in front of like a thousand people. It's a big deal. Some pretty famous people have won it, including Bob Dole and that hiker who had to cut off his arm to free himself from underneath a boulder [Aron Ralston]."

"Yeah . . ." Jeff said.

"I was just calling to let you know that the person who won that award this year . . . is you."

"What?" Jeff said. "What did you say?"

"I said I nominated you for this national award—the Shining Star of Perseverance—and you won. It's going to be really nice. They're going to fly you and Deb to Kansas City and put you up at the Hyatt."

"Are you kidding?"

"No. They're going to take you to a fancy dinner, you're going to get to throw out the first pitch at a Kansas City Royals baseball game."

"Are you *serious*?"

"Yeah. And they're going to honor you at a huge ceremony in front of like a thousand people."

Jeff took his foot off his desk and sat up at attention. "I . . . am . . . *speechless*!" he said. "Thank you a million times isn't enough. I mean, just for the nomination, let alone winning the award! I won the award?"

"You sure did, partner," I said. "And nobody deserves it more."

"Thank you!" he repeated. "This is . . . unbelievable!"

Jeff had won prestigious awards before. About two months after his miracle, John Carroll University presented him with the Campion Shield for Heroism, an award that had been given to only two other people in the school's one-hundred-year history. That meant a lot. But nothing meant more to him than this national award for perseverance.

When he hung up the phone, he walked upstairs to his bedroom, where Debra was folding laundry. He tried to be cool but couldn't pull it off. He looked at his wife with a huge grin. "What's going on?" she said in a suspicious voice.

"Oh, I was just chatting with Jim," he said. "We were talking about the book. Turns out that things are progressing pretty well, and that . . . we're going to be going to Kansas City!"

"What?" Debra said.

"And we're not going to Jim's home, either, to visit."

Debra's face froze as she waited for details.

"Unknown to me, Jim nominated me for a national perseverance award, and guess who your winner is?"

"No way!" Debra screamed. "A *national* award?" She gave him a big hug and pushed the clothes aside that were on the bed. "Sit down and tell me about it."

Several days later John called and told me Assurant wanted to give Jeff a surprise—his own authentic Royals jersey complete with his name on the back. "They want to know what number he'd like on the jersey," John said.

I couldn't ask Jeff so I called Debra, who then called Jeff's dad. "Thirty-four would be a good number, because on March 4, 2004, we 'marched forth' into a new life!" he said, referring to the day Jeff's batteries were turned on. Thirty-four also was the number of Jeff's favorite sports hero—the late Walter Payton, Hall of Fame running back for the Chicago Bears.

It was *perfect*. Jeff was going to flip!

Jeff and Debra flew to Kansas City on Monday, July 24. He called me when he got into town.

I had some fun with him. "Mr. Matovic," I said. "I'm a scout for the Kansas City Royals. I hear you're a lanky fireballer who's going to be throwing out the first pitch tonight. I want you to keep warm. We may just need you later in the game." He laughed.

The first night Assurant honored him with a dinner. About twenty people attended. We all ate at Pierpont's, an upscale steak restaurant inside Kansas City's historic Union Station. The place was fancy and impressive, with dark wood and a huge wine storage rack. It was so dimly lit I could hardly see the menu. Jeff wore a dark suit, and Debra a pretty dress.

Steve Palermo, a deeply tan, highly regarded former Major League Baseball umpire and bona fide hero who was shot and paralyzed in 1991 attempting to foil a robbery, commanded the room with confidence and charisma. But with Palermo as his biggest cheerleader, Jeff became the star of the dinner, answering questions and enthralling everyone with stories from his life.

Next came the award ceremony, during which Jeff received the award and spoke in front of a thousand people in a downtown banquet hall.

Steve Palermo put it best: "Through this award," he said, "Jeff Matovic will serve as a beacon of hope to others fighting to overcome obstacles, and as an example to all that obstacles need not be insurmountable."

Jeff beamed as he accepted the award and received his surprise— an official number 34 Royals jersey with his name on the back which he slipped into in front of the cheering crowd.

Moments earlier, he had given his speech:

The Shining Star of Perseverance Award means a great deal to me, for its representation transcends many different horizons and crosses countless boundaries. One may look at this award as a token of appreciation for all I have been fortunate enough to endure and fight for. In reality, your presence here today, along with my loving wife, Debra, is a true representation of how I view this great honor. My new lease on life takes place not in the past on February 9, when micro-sized electrodes were placed deep within my brain. Nor was it February 20, 2004, the day that doctors Robert Maciunas and Brian Maddux provided me with a gift nothing short of miraculous. The true miracle of my deep brain stimulation surgery takes place each and every day when I awaken to stillness and a world of opportunity that I have been dreaming of since the age of three.

Since the beauty of stillness embraced my body on March 4, 2004, I have come to realize numerous facts that do not lie or deceive, but rather deposit truth where truth is needed most. Truth cannot be spotted on the exterior of a person, in a crowded room, or even where best of friends sit and reminisce about times gone by. I believe that we live truth—day in and day out. Thesauruses provide alternate words to tell us about truth—reality, actuality, unvarnished, unmasked, authentic, genuine, and sincere. One may ask what I found common among all these meanings that assist me in my journey. The answer lies not in a riddle or puzzle, nor in a chest with a combination lock. What many people take for granted, as I did prior to March 4, is the fact that if we look hard enough, truth stares us right in the eye. Truth is a governing principle of life. Much like a compass will show us true north, truth will guide our hearts, minds, and souls to where we need to be, not where we want to be.

Tourette Syndrome placed many obstacles in my way throughout the last thirty-three years. Some of these barriers I found too solid to break; others were easier, while others were worse than I could imagine. How I got through the labyrinth of confusion only to arrive in the care of a wonderful surgical team at the University Hospitals of Cleveland often baffles me. However, through this thirty-three-year battle, one truth that I held certain and dear to my heart, as I do now, is a relentless pursuit to be me. Not rich, athletically gifted, an A-plus student, nor an owner of priceless gold treasures, I wanted only to release the gifts God gave me that were trapped inside of a dark cage with no known key.

Many of you may have heard of the late, great NFL running back Walter Payton. I grew up admiring Walter for his incredible athletic moves, blazing speed, and heroic agility when the game was on the line. But what I always will remember about this man are the following: One, that he was told that he would never have a shot at being drafted into the NFL due to his five-foot-ten, slender frame; two, he was not going to make it big because he was not from a university that received weekly national attention; three, it was not in the cards for him to even begin to compete in the National Football League because his overall presence was not intimidating and fearful.

But what I saw in Walter was what I began to see in myself: an untiring and unwavering work ethic, with resilience to obstacles and a passion to succeed. Unyielding willpower and faith were the attributes that made him one of the best running backs in the history of the National Football League. His family surrounded him and embraced him for who he was: his size, abilities, and areas for opportunity.

Friends helped Walter to make the most out of each day. Although I will never possess his vision for heroic running on the football field, we do share a very common and unbreakable thread. As Walter used to say, "I will not be held back by lack of size or strength. I will conquer my enemies on and off the field by running around them, over them, or by plowing straight through them." His authentic belief in his own abilities was the component that made him a man of integrity on and off the field.

Nobody can ever measure the heart of a champion. And for Walter's teachings, even though he didn't know I was watching and taking mental notes, I am eternally grateful. For these are the principles that guided me to tackle my own demons and eventually find that hidden key to unlock the potential inside.

When faced with the adversity and stress of everyday life, I hope to be a beacon of light, hope, and strength when individuals and families cannot find the path they seek. My deep brain stimulation surgery has yielded wonderful results for my family and I. More important, I hope that the recognition that this procedure has brought to Tourette Syndrome and neurological research will invoke continued belief and encouragement. With our combined efforts, we can make Tourette Syndrome a household phrase that is understood, respected, and pursued with medical research.

Although I guard and value the stillness of life, the graduate and doctoral program within which I have reengaged, and the opportunities to soon enter the corporate world, these are not at the heart of what life is all about.

Life is special now because of the ability to walk through a mall without laughing gestures being thrown my way. Life is the morning calls of "Daddy" coming from my twenty-month-old child, Christopher, who, without the miracle of this surgery, would not be here today. Life is the ability to look someone in the eye and converse and then calmly extend my hand to shake theirs. Life is about being able to drink out of a glass instead of a plastic sipper cup. Life is my family—my wife, Debra; my daughter, Bonnie; and sons, Michael and Christopher.

My life is surrounded by family and friends who have believed in the same dream that has brought me to be with you today. Without the tireless efforts and sacrifices from my parents, Jim and Patty; and brother, Steve; and his wife, Lisa, life would not have had the same meaning. They have researched Tourette Syndrome, driven to countless doctor appointments, cried with me, and tried to find some meaning among all the madness this disorder brings. I will forever be indebted to them for sacrificing themselves for the betterment of me. Many friends have also shared my belief and walked beside me. Jay, Paul, Joe, and our very good friends who are present with us today, Jim and Susan Fussell, have given more of themselves than they realize.

Life is astoundingly present, colorful, and exciting for someone like myself who has sought what others view as "regular, routine, and simple." Through the will to persevere and combat obstacles that invaded my life, I am filled with joy as individuals worldwide have called, e-mailed, and sent letters to thank my family and I for the hope we have given. Calls received from Canada, the UK, Australia, Germany, South Africa, and the United States have given me strength to keep fighting for the insightful research that is due for Tourette Syndrome.

With ambitious technique, my life goals are now steered in two specific directions: [first] to provide support and education to individuals and families suffering from Tourette Syndrome. This support comes in the form of public speaking at universities, clinics, support-group gatherings, and phone conversations. The second direction is the attainment of my master's degree in psychology, where I am currently specializing in the counseling and treatment of mental health disorders with concentrations in pediatric and family Tourette Syndrome and stress management techniques. With these two goals lining my new life path, I have found what I know to be a virtuous truth and a welcome opportunity to serve others.

Thus far, my public speaking has provided me with an opportunity to share similarities and differences with other members of the community with various disorders. These interactions not only provide strength and encouragement for me, but also assist in the feedback to others who, much like myself, have found particular struggles along the path of life. Along with greater Kansas City and surrounding communities, the world seeks a better quality of life for those that suffer from any disability.

Regardless of symptoms, diagnosis, or prognosis, we all share a common lifeline and a common bond. We are all a part of a unique and honorable community in which we are free to live— free to live our dreams, regardless of what others say or think. We are bound by nothing. We are free to imagine. Exploration in diversity is a shared strength as we lift each other up and together celebrate the Shining Star of Perseverance award.

Oliver Wendell Holmes [once said], "A moment's insight is sometimes worth a life's experience." I have found truth in this statement and furthermore have gained a sense of being, regardless of what the world tells us we should be. Like Walter Payton, I chose to run around, through, or over the obstacles that I faced. I remained determined and focused to let my commitment shine forth to eventually conquer Tourette Syndrome. My refusal to accept physical and mental limitations has not only brought my family and I a new lease on life and an extraordinary sense of group accomplishment, but has given me direction and purpose.

To win any war, even those within ourselves, we need to fight the battles. And much like the soft-flowing stream that eventually erodes the rock in its way, we must keep fighting and believing— in ourselves and others, all the while knowing we are not alone.

Perseverance has brought me peace, well-being, and a sense of direction. May the acceptance of this award today be a shared insight among all of us so that together we may find a clear sense of experience and live the dream that awaits us all.

My special thanks are offered to the WillReturn Council of Assurant Employee Benefits as I am honored to be the recipient of such a prestigious award. May your contributions to the community find you personal and professional feelings of accomplishment and gratification. And for all your efforts to assist individuals in need, may you find resilience to obstacles, proactivity within what is truth, conscientiousness in living in the moment, and willpower to remain strong and determined as you already are.

He received a standing ovation.

— ▬ —

AS GREAT AS the first two events were, the third was even better. That was the night Jeff got to live out a childhood dream as the Royals played host to the Baltimore Orioles.

Before the game, while the crew prepared the field, Steve Palermo took Jeff and Assurant vice president Mark Bohen onto the field. They talked and took pictures in front of the Royals dugout. Jeff looked like a Royals pitcher in his white and blue Royals jersey. A team official acted excited when he saw him.

"Are you a lefty?" he asked.

"Sorry," Jeff answered.

"Dang," he said with a smile.

Mark Bohen smacked a fist into his catcher's mitt. "I haven't caught a ball in eight years," he said. "So don't do anything crazy."

"Well I haven't thrown one in a while, so I'm just hoping I don't get it dirty," Jeff replied.

Palermo turned to Jeff. "You got the balls to stand on the mound, or are you going to stand in front of it?" he said.

"Are you kidding me?" Jeff said, staring at the ball. "I grew up playing sports all my life. This is a dream come true! And if you think I am skipping being on that mound to throw an actual major league pitch, you've got to be *crazy*!"

Before Jeff knew it, the moment had arrived. People started filing into the seats at Kauffman Stadium. He got the signal, and he and Mark smiled at each other and prepared to walk onto the field.

"Tonight's ceremonial first pitch is being thrown by Jeff Matovic of Cleveland, Ohio, who was just awarded the Shining Star of Perseverance award given by the WillReturn Council in recognition of overcoming a lifelong disorder. Please help me welcome . . . Jeff Matovic."

Jeff and Mark walked onto the field and stopped on the first-baseline to wave to the crowd. Then Bohen walked to the plate as Jeff headed slowly for the mound. He wanted to take every step as slowly as possible. As he walked he couldn't help indulging his fantasy. In his head he imagined a deep voice echoing through the stadium.

Now pitching for the Kansas City Royals, number thirty-four, Jeff Matovic!

When he finally reached the mound, he was in no hurry to look at home plate. He looked around first. The pitching rubber was a perfect white as he touched it with his right shoe.

I cannot believe what I am about to do, he thought as he gazed around the cavernous stadium.

"God," he said, "thank you so much for granting me this moment." He needed to turn around for the pitch. Then he remembered. He had always promised himself if he ever got the chance to be on a professional mound that he was going to see just how big the outfield was.

There's so much open space out there, he'd think when he watched baseball on TV. *And you can't find a place to get a hit?*

Jeff motioned to Bohen by raising a finger on his left hand as if to say "one moment" then turned toward the sun to gaze into the outfield. It was indeed enormous. Instantly he gained an appreciation for how fast, and how good, major league outfielders were. He imagined a *SportsCenter* highlight with an outfielder tracking down a well-hit ball.

Are you serious? he thought. *He's got to cover that much ground? He better be a track sprinter too!*

Then he turned back around. Time for the pitch. Just outside of Assurant's suite, I shouted my approval. "Yeah, Jeff!" I shouted, cupping my hands and yelling at loudly as I could.

He pointed to me in the stands. And for one brief moment he felt like a real major leaguer who had a fan. He locked onto Mark with the ball behind his back. When I saw him step back and go into his windup, everything seemed to go in slow motion. I couldn't hear anything. It was just him, on the mound, in one of the prettiest stadiums in the major leagues.

He delivered the pitch, a little outside the left edge of the plate and thrown purposely high to ensure the ball would not get dirty. After

Mark caught it, he jogged out to the mound as if Jeff had just struck out the last batter in the bottom of the ninth. He stuck out his hand and patted Jeff on the shoulder, then handed him the ball as they jogged into the Royals dugout, waving to the crowd.

Later, in the suite, Jeff asked Palermo—if it wouldn't be too much trouble—if he could get a ball signed by the team. "That would mean a tremendous amount to me," he said.

"I'll try," Palermo replied.

After twenty minutes Palermo returned to the suite. He walked up to Jeff with a goofy smirk and his hands behind his back, nodding his head. "Enjoying that food there?" he said.

Jeff nodded.

"Regarding that baseball that you wanted me to have signed by the Royals team—" he said.

Oh my God, Jeff thought. *Was he able to pull that off?*

"I wasn't able to do that," he said, "but I was hanging around a guy named Brett shootin' the shit, and . . ." He held up a brand-new major league baseball with a perfect George Brett signature in blue ink.

"You've heard of this guy, right?"

"Heard of him?" Jeff said. "He's a legend!"

Jeff gave him a hug.

"Steve, this means more than you can possibly imagine!" he said. "I will *always* treasure this. It will be put in a case above my desk. I'll tell stories for decades about this ball and our time together."

At the end of the game, which the Royals won, Palermo bearhugged Jeff before we left the suite. They had talked all night. Bonded. You could tell Palermo respected Jeff, even *admired* him. Before we left he held Jeff closely in a manly embrace and spoke softly in his ear.

"As Mike Ditka once told me, you got the balls of a lion, kid. The balls of a lion!"

47

"What Do You Mean I Won?"

THE YEARS AFTER Jeff's award went quickly. I worked at the *Star* during the day, and at night I worked on the book, often calling Jeff to interview. It wasn't easy. I was *so tired*, and I seemingly hurt more with every passing day.

In many ways I lived for Jeff and the promise of our book. And every day there was one thought that kept me going: if Jeff had the courage to survive what he had survived, certainly I could endure whatever hardships I had to face.

He was my hero and my inspiration. And in July of 2009, I found out just how much that inspiration meant to me.

❦

THE CALL CAME early to my office, and I was in no mood to take it. Exhausted and trying to finish a long story on deadline, the last thing I wanted to do was talk to someone. That's why when the phone rang at my desk I almost didn't answer it.

"The *Kansas City Star*, go away," I said picking up the receiver without pressing the answer button. I imagined I had heat-ray vision that melted it into a small, beige lump. Unfortunately the lump kept ringing. I sighed, rolled my eyes, and answered it for real.

"The *Kansas City Star.* This is Jim Fussell speaking. May I help you?" I said in an uninspired voice. The woman on the other end of the line was like no one I typically heard from. She didn't sound like an editor, a reader, a PR flak, or a source. She was cheery—*oddly cheery* for that early in the morning. The woman had a high, excited voice and she was talking fast, congratulating me on winning this or that from the ' American association of something or other.

I tried to slow her down. "Wait . . ." I said. "Whoa. What?"

She kept talking. And while I'm sure she was a fine person, her cheeriness was off-putting. Who was *that* happy *that early* in the morning?

"I'm sorry," I said, interrupting her gleeful prattling. "What's this all about again?"

"You won!" she said, her voice nearly rising into a squeal. "You won first place!"

"Wait," I said. "*What* won?"

"Your story!" she said. "It won first place in the American Association of Sunday and Feature Editors [now called the Society for Features Journalism] writing contest."

I laughed. I would have *loved* to believe that was true. I didn't. It was a mistake. She had a wrong number. "Look," I said, "you sound like a very nice woman. But you must have the wrong person. I don't enter writing contests."

"Is this . . . James A. Fussell of the *Kansas City Star*?"

"Uh-huh."

"Well then you *won*!" she said, her voice rising again into a giddy squeak. "Congratulations! And this is a *big one*, for general feature. This is the one *everyone* wants to win!"

"But—I didn't *enter* anything," I protested.

"Well, someone must have entered it for you," the woman said. "Because here it is. And here you are. And *you won*! Congratulations!"

"Wait. What story are you talking about?"

"Uhh, it's right here." She read the headline. "One Who Has Lived the Life Becomes Agent of Change."

"Oh, the story about Kristy Childs and Veronica's Voice?" I said. Silence.

"The prostitute-with-a-heart-of-gold story?"

"Yes! That's the one," she said. "It was an excellent story."

"Somebody entered that?" I said.

"Apparently so. And it won!"

"Well that's *great news*!" I said, genuinely shocked. "Uhh, thank you!"

We talked for several more minutes about the story, the contest, and the upcoming convention in Portland, Oregon.

I smiled broadly when I hung up the phone. I had won a *national award*—one a lot of others apparently wanted to win. Not only that, I had won it at the highest level, competing against reporters at such venerable papers as the *New York Times*, the *Washington Post*, and the *Wall Street Journal.*

I laughed at the thought. *Me?* Unreal.

It must have been the subject. The woman I had written about— Kristy Childs—certainly was an impressive person. A former prostitute with a harrowing background, she had founded Veronica's Voice, a Kansas City group that hit the streets after dark to help women leave the life. I had fought for the story and for the time needed to do it right. It took many months of hard work. Persuading prostitutes they could trust me was not something I rushed. I remember working late many nights to rewrite it and fine-tune it to get it right. Turns out my editor at the time, David Frese—who was a huge help in structuring the story and making it better—had entered the story for me and never told me. I walked to his desk and thanked him.

"Hey, it was your story, man," he said.

"Yeah. But it wouldn't have been as good without your help. And it certainly couldn't have won if you hadn't have entered it. I want you to know how much both of those things mean to me."

"Happy to do it," he said. "It was a fantastic story."

"Thank you," I said.

But there was someone else I needed to thank. I never would have had the energy or drive to complete such a long and difficult piece of reporting and writing without the inspiration I got from Jeff's miracle.

That evening I called Jeff and told him the news. "There's a prestigious national award given every year by the American Association of Sunday and Feature Editors that honors the best-written feature story of the year at all the biggest papers in the United States and Canada," I said. "Uhh . . . guess who just won it this year?"

"You're kidding!" he said.

"Nope."

"You?"

"Hard to believe, isn't it?"

"Not at all," he said. "That's fantastic, Jim!" he said. "Congratulations!"

"Thank you," I said. "But here's the best part. They honor the winners in Portland this year, and I've decided that . . . I'm going. And since I couldn't have done this without you, I want you to come with me."

I didn't hear anything for several seconds.

"Are you kidding me?" he said. "I don't know what to say."

"Say you'll be my guest," I said.

"Absolutely," he said, laughing in disbelief. "I'd be honored!"

48

Revenge of the Weirdos

SITTING ON THE bed in my well-appointed hotel room in Portland, Oregon, I twisted my back until my vertebrae cracked like a piece of twisted bubble wrap. I wasn't twenty anymore. But on this day, fifty-one felt more like eighty-one.

It was September 2009. I had come to Portland as one of a handful of newspaper writers and editors who were being honored at a prestigious national journalism conference. Since the conference didn't officially start until tomorrow, I had time to goof around. I removed my athletic socks and rolled them into little white balls. Spotting a black wastebasket in the corner of the room, I began bobbing like a point guard looking for his shot.

Fussell at the top of the key, down one with five seconds to go. Fakes left, goes right. Wants the lane but is cut off. Three, two, he's in trouble. Throws up a prayer...

The wobbly sock ball arced high in the air, kissed softly off the side of the wall, then dropped in the waste can with a satisfying thunk.

It's gooooood!

I bounded off the bed and gave myself a high five as I did a little victory dance and sashayed into the bathroom. That is, until I became light-headed and had to lean against the sink until the room stopped spinning. I was just tired from the trip, I told myself.

I knew better. I shook my head, and a familiar pain shot through my neck and radiated down my back. For a moment I felt like I was going to collapse. Biting hard on my lip, I shut my eyes and grimaced until the feeling passed.

I needed to soak in a hot bath. I turned on the water and got undressed. As the tub filled I pulled on an overly fluffy hotel bathrobe and walked to the corner to fish my sock out of the trash can. Tossing the sock on my open suitcase, I sat down at the small desk to start a trip journal on my laptop.

> Sept. 23, 2009: After five hours of flying I feel like my head is going to explode. My hotel seems nice, but I haven't had a chance to look around much. Probably go down to the lobby and check things out before the conference starts at 7. Jeff's plane arrives tonight close to midnight. Must have polished his watch a dozen times already.

By now I could see wisps of steam wafting into the main room.

"You're bath is ready, sir," I said in a stuffy English accent. As I turned the corner to the bathroom the moist air hit me in the face like a hot towel. Standing over the tub, I tested the temperature by dipping my big toe in the water.

"Holy shit!" I said, yanking my foot from the tub so fast I nearly fell in the toilet. It's not like I had to go the burn unit or anything, but now my big toe looked like a radish.

I drained several inches of scalding water, then ran some cold before mixing it vigorously with large, sweeping loops of my arm. A twinge shot up my right side as if I had been shot. I dipped my other big toe in the water, this time with a more satisfying result. Letting the robe drop, I submerged myself in a warm, wet cocoon. My entire body sunk under the water, save for the top part of my mouth, which stuck from the surface like the blowhole of a whale. When the hot water cooled, I added more.

An hour later, the bath had done its job. I was so relaxed when I stepped out, I didn't even bother to dry off. I just stood there dripping onto a white bath towel.

Naked and soaking, I wiped the condensation off the mirror and gazed into my bloodshot blue eyes. Fifteen hundred miles from home,

I watched as I moved my head to the left and then slowly back to the right. I took a deep breath and stared at myself as I counted backward from one hundred. No pain. No tightness. Why couldn't I just *freeze* like this? God, Tourette Syndrome sucked.

"Eighty-nine, eighty-eight . . ." And then those familiar feelings returned—the slowly building pressure, the unbearable stress, the all-consuming desire to *shake the hell out of my head.*

"Focus," I said. "Don't move." And for a while I didn't.

"Fifty-five, fifty-four."

But when I reached thirty I couldn't stand it any more. I moved my head slowly to the left, then wrenched it violently back to the right. I shook it so hard my wet hair flung a small shower of water droplets around the room—so hard I nearly knocked myself to the floor. Temporarily out of breath, I bent over and grabbed my knees. A jolt of electric pain flashed across the muscles of my upper back as a wave of dizziness blasted through my brain. When I stood up I caught sight of myself in the hazy, water-spotted mirror, a pained expression on my face.

"Hello, weirdo," I said.

"No," I immediately corrected myself. "Not today. You're *more* than that."

I smiled and moved closer to the mirror until my nose almost touched the glass. "You hear me?" I nodded, and gave myself a soft pat on the back.

After getting dressed, I grabbed my laptop and headed for the lobby. I still had several hours to kill before the conference's opening reception, and I needed to get used to being around large groups of people again.

The lobby was crowded, and I began to feel uncomfortable almost immediately after stepping off the elevator. I found a bathroom and ducked in to splash some cold water on my face. Looking in the mirror I smiled at myself, as if that would make the deep bags under my eyes disappear. It did, but who was I kidding? I was just trading dark eye circles for crooked, yellow teeth. At least the water felt good. I dried my brown goatee with a swipe of my hand, and used the wetness to sweep my straight brown hair to the side. I took a deep breath. I had just about steeled myself for reentering the lobby when a teenager with long hair and a tattoo of Bob Marley on his arm walked a little too closely to me at the sink. I blinked three times and twitched as if poked by a cattle prod.

"Dude," he said, edging away. "That's messed up."

"That's an interesting way to put it," I said. "But yes it is. Thanks for noticing."

When I was finally ready to leave the bathroom, I saw dozens of people milling around the lobby who looked very much like they belonged at a journalism conference. Many carried newspapers or wrote on computers. I found a good spot in an out-of-the-way place and opened my laptop, hoping to fit in. I sat on an antique, caramel-colored couch in jeans and a black linen shirt. I had my reading glasses on top of my head, a blue pen tucked behind one ear, and a long black comb balanced behind the other. As I began to write, a man vaguely resembling actor Christian Slater (who I later learned was restaurant manager Nick Stoddart) approached in a black tuxedo carrying a silver tray of food.

"Good evening, sir," he said in a voice worthy of a character from an old movie. "May I interest you in some foie gras? It's served on a toasted brioche point with a grilled Bosc pear, a garnish of tomato-fig marmalade, and a chive spear."

I looked up from my screen and wrinkled my nose. "I'm not sure I'm *classy* enough for foie gras," I said, trying my best to hide the fact that I couldn't quite remember what foie gras was.

He recoiled at the possibility. "Of course you are, sir," he said. "You're sitting in the Benson."

He had a point. The Benson was a one-hundred-year-old grand hotel on the National Register of Historic Places. Simon Benson, a lumber baron, spared no expense. He spent a million dollars to build and furnish the place in 1912 at a time when a worker's average yearly salary was $646.

A cast-iron railing escorted visitors up an Italian marble staircase, and dozens of Austrian-crystal chandeliers hung from the classically coffered ceiling. The wood used to make the walls and soaring square pillars in the lobby were fashioned from Circassian walnut bought from Czar Nicholas II and imported from the forests of imperial Russia. Every president since William Howard Taft had slept in its presidential suite. The place just smelled rich.

I smiled and took some foie gras.

Besides, maybe I was classier than I thought. I pulled a real gold one-hundred-year-old pocket watch from my laptop bag. The twenty-four-jewel double roller seemed right at home in the elegant lobby of the Benson. And soon, so did I.

Until I lost my comb.

I don't go *anywhere* without my long black comb. When I comb my hair with it, or balance it behind my ear, it makes me feel more comfortable. Linus had his blanket; I have my comb.

All of which explains why I started to panic when I couldn't find it. A wave of discomfort seized control of my head, cocking it like a gun. And just when I thought I couldn't stand it anymore, I heard a voice.

"I think this is yours." I looked up to see an older, white-haired woman in a red dress, my comb extended from her hand like a wand.

"It is," I sighed. "Thank you." Relieved, I slumped back onto the couch, breathing hard.

"Are you OK?" she asked.

"Yeah," I said. "Well, no. . . . But yeah."

The woman looked confused.

"Jim," I said, extending my hand.

"Ella," she said, grasping it.

We talked for a while—about the comb, the conference, and Jeff and the book.

"Why do you call him a miracle man?" she asked.

I laughed. "How much time ya got?"

"My daughter won't be here for hours," she said.

I took a long breath and finished the last of my foie gras, which was surprisingly good considering I finally remembered it was duck liver. Then I told Ella the story from beginning to end.

After I finished, she thanked me for sharing. "That's *wonderful!*" she said, wearing the smile of someone who had just been given a special gift. It made me feel so good that she reacted that way to our story and gave me hope that others might feel the same way.

I tried to go back to writing but there were too many distractions. I excused myself and walked several blocks from the hotel to a group of downtown street vendors to buy dinner—a saucy pork and rice dish that I took back to my room.

Later, close to midnight, I climbed into my rented white Nissan Altima to pick up Jeff at Portland International. I rubbed my neck as I walked through the large, clean terminal to Jeff's gate. I should have been tired, but the closer I got, the more energized I felt. I began thinking of all the things Jeff and I had done and all that he had meant to me.

Scanning the passengers as they walked off the plane, I spotted his smiling face immediately as he walked toward me in a peach-colored shirt.

"Howdy, stranger," he said. "I just came here because I heard something about someone being a national award winner?"

"That's funny," I said. " 'Cause I heard the same thing about you."

Jeff smiled. "How ya doing, partner?"

"Can't complain for after midnight," I said.

We talked about everything and nothing as we drove back to the Benson. We should have gotten some rest, but we were too excited. Besides, Jeff was starving. We decided to go out and see what Portland had to offer after hours in its well-designed downtown.

It was a perfect night—warm and still. We wandered the downtown streets after midnight, amazed at how dramatically life could turn around. Five years ago we were both at our lowest points and didn't even know each other. Now we were best friends, he had his Tourette's under control, we had both won national awards, and we were writing a book together.

Well after 1:00 AM we stopped in a corner bar and sat down.

"Kitchen still open?" I asked the man behind the bar.

"Absolutely," he said.

We ordered cheeseburgers and fries. We were the only ones in the place. It had wood paneling and an open, airy feeling, as if you were sitting outside. I wanted to remember this moment forever. I was glad Jeff was there with me. We had come through so much. And now our amazing, unlikely journey was unfolding, and finishing, right in front of our eyes in the middle of the night in Portland, Oregon.

"This is all so surreal," I said.

Jeff raised his glass. "Well, you *are* a national award winner," he said.

"And so are you," I said with a grin. We clinked glasses.

We polished off the last fry and headed out. Still hungry, we continued walking toward a local landmark I'd been told we had to visit—Voodoo Doughnut. The place was famous for its unusual dough-nuts, eclectic décor, and iconic pink boxes that carried the company's logo and drawings of voodoo priests.

We finally made it to the place, but only after stepping over several vagrants who were passed out on the sidewalk in front of us. The place was packed with college students and seemingly every tattooed, blue-haired, exotically pierced, countercultural character Portland had to offer. The line was out the door and around the block.

We laughed as we talked with strangers, hearing their stories and telling them ours. For two grown men well out of college, this was a ton of fun. We finally made it into the store, which smelled amazing. We laughed at signs that read: I GOT VD IN PORTLAND, and THE MAGIC IS IN THE HOLE! Inside glass cases the one-of-a-kind doughnuts were as odd and unusual as the people in line, including several pornographically shaped ones and others that defied easy description. We knew what we wanted: one of the place's specialties that had been recommended to us in line by several of the characters: the maple bacon!

We ordered two of the maple bars that were topped with crispy strips of bacon, and smiled all the way back to our hotel. Back at the Benson, we paused to take in the extraordinary scenery. For two more hours we strolled the grounds of the historic hotel, appreciating our surroundings.

"This is fantastic!" Jeff said of the opulent decor. "Oh, Deb would *love* this!"

We even met the restaurant manager, Nick Stoddart, and got a personal tour of the Benson's restaurant. Standing by a table next to a wall, Nick stopped.

"You want to see something?" he said.

We nodded our heads.

Before we knew it Nick did something that caused a portion of the wall to open, allowing us access to one of the coolest wine cellars we had ever seen. The place was like the Bat Cave, only stocked with wine. It was old, and cold, and felt oddly like it could be haunted.

It was nearing 4:00 AM. We asked Nick to take our picture in the cellar before finally calling it a night.

THE NEXT DAY we got dressed up for the awards banquet. The lunchtime buffet was like everything else in the hotel—first class. Everything—from the seafood and the mountains of fresh fruits to the Kobe beef sliders and endless desserts—couldn't have been better. We sat at a table with other award recipients from around the country and Mary Lou Nolan, an assistant managing editor from the *Star*.

When my name was called as the winner of general feature—one of the most prestigious awards—it was one of the proudest moments of my life. There I was, in the middle of some of the top reporters in the country, including Pulitzer Prize winners and writers from influential papers such as the *New York Times*, the *Washington Post*, and the *Wall Street Journal*. And when they called the name of the winner of the best general feature story that year—anywhere in the United States or Canada—it was *my name* they called.

A chill ran through my body as I walked to the front to accept the plaque. I tried to walk as slowly as I could, trying to make the moment last forever.

This was a miracle if I had ever seen one. A miracle of my very own. I won the award. Me—the guy who shakes his head and cries under his desk and hurts so much he wonders if he will have the strength to go on.

Are you serious?

I smiled as I held the award up and briefly pointed toward Jeff on the way back to my seat. Back at the table, Jeff passed me a note, telling me he couldn't have been more proud of me. *No*, I kept thinking, *I couldn't have done this without* you.

That evening I took Jeff out for a celebratory steak dinner to tell him that. We walked several blocks to Ruth's Chris Steak House and ordered some of the best beef I have ever tasted. Jeff also got some complimentary shrimp, which melted in his mouth. It was perfect end to a perfect day—and the best time to show Jeff how much his amazing life had inspired me.

"I can't tell you how much your story of courage and bravery has meant to me in my life," I told him. "It has helped give me back my hope, and helped me to take on larger stories that I wouldn't have had the energy to tackle before. You helped me believe again in the power of miracles. And for that I will never be able to thank you enough."

I took the shiny gold pocket watch from my bag and handed it to him. "But maybe this will say what I can't."

"Oh my God, Jim," he said, cradling the watch in his large hands. "This is *beautiful*. Are you sure this is for me?"

"Absolutely," I said.

"Wow," he said, temporarily at a loss for words. "I mean . . . this is one of the nicest things anyone has ever done for me."

"Turn it over," I said.

He flipped over the one-hundred-year-old antique and read the inscription on the back.

"Just remember," he read. "You are a man for others . . . a miracle man!"

"I couldn't have done this without you," I said. "We would not be sitting here right now without you. So thank you. Thank you *so much*."

"Thank you!" Jeff said, shaking his head.

Suddenly the whole story made sense to me. And for the first time I understood my place in it when it came to the book. This was the last piece to the puzzle, both a perfect ending and a beginning to the book we'd been working on for years. It was Jeff's story. It was my story. But most of all, it was *our* story. It was Me—and the Miracle Man.

I laughed at the elegant simplicity of it all. After all we had been through, we had come out the other side better for it. We had found each other and found a purpose in our story. This felt like victory, and not just because of my award. It was the sum total of everything we had accomplished together. And it was easily one of the happiest moments of my life.

I looked across the table at my partner, my brother, my hero, and raised my glass high in the air.

"You know something," I said, as we clinked glasses, "for a couple of weirdos with Tourette Syndrome, we're not doing too badly."

Epilogue

WRITING THIS BOOK was the single hardest thing I've ever done—and the most rewarding. I started it nine years ago with a man I didn't know. Along the way he became my hero, my friend, and the brother I never had. We collaborated as partners. Through the experience we learned that *nothing* is impossible with enough passion, perseverance, and hard work.

The book did not end up in the same place it began. We started with Jeff's miracle, which was incredible on its own. The more we talked about our Tourette's the more we became entwined in each other's lives and the more we realized that this story was a living thing—organic and changing. It was Jeff's story, mixed with my story, that became *our* story. It was a journey of discovery, an open-ended tale of one miracle that spawned several others.

If you learn anything from this book, let it be this: your problems are only the difficulties you can see now. Even if they seem insurmountable, don't give up. You have *no idea* how things may change tomorrow, or what's just around the corner. But more than that, realize that no matter who you are or what you're going through, like Jeff you have the capacity to inspire others and change lives with nothing more than sheer willpower and a caring heart.

Many things have happened since the completion of this book. Today—thanks in part to the courage of Jeff Matovic and the skill of Dr. Robert Maciunas and Dr. Brian Maddux—deep brain stimulation surgeries are being done around the globe in greater numbers, giving hope of relief to patients with the most severe cases of Tourette Syndrome.

On a personal note, Jeff and I dream of being a motivational speaking team. Thanks to his miraculous surgery and the effect it has had on me, that's actually possible.

Debra and Susan continue to be the best wives and mothers around. We are truly blessed to have them in our lives, because the truth is we wouldn't have survived without them.

Today, several years after his surgery, Jeff continues to enjoy a life free of tics. He is determined to take advantage of the opportunity he's been given. Currently he is working as an academic tutor and motivational speaker. It is important to note that while his tics are completely controlled, he is not cured. He will be free of tics as long as the stimulator in his brain and the batteries in his chest continue to work. Every three to five years his batteries must be replaced in a small outpatient surgery. It's a small price to pay for getting your life back.

Shortly after his operation, University Hospitals Case Medical Center received a multimillion-dollar grant to study the use of deep brain stimulation in people with severe Tourette Syndrome. Hundreds of patients from all over the world applied, many making emotional pleas about their dire situation or that of a loved one. Doctors evaluated all the applications, then chose eight patients for the first phase of the trial. While not all surgeries were 100 percent successful, five patients experienced a life-changing reduction or elimination of their tics. This first-of-its-kind study determined that DBS can reduce tic frequency and severity in some adults who have exhausted other medical treatments.

In addition to patients who got help through the clinical trials, countless others have been inspired to write or call Jeff and Debra, expressing their admiration and thanks for the courage and determination it took to endure this suffering and find a way to triumph over it.

Jeff and Debra continue to live in Cleveland and have added another new member to their family—their second son, Andy—bringing the number of their children to four. The two younger boys are rambunctious and full of energy and show all the signs of being tall, good-looking athletes like their father. Their son Chris, the older of the two, was born one year to the day after Dr. Maciunas said yes to doing deep brain stimulation for Jeff. Not to be outdone, Andy was born on the three-year anniversary of Jeff's February 9 miracle surgery. Debra's older children, Bonnie and Mike, are now young adults in college looking forward to bright futures.

As for me, I am still at the *Kansas City Star.* Susan and I will soon celebrate our thirty-third wedding anniversary. Our daughter, Allison, has gone off to the University of Kansas, while our older son, Patrick, is living in Lawrence, Kansas, where he is pursuing a life in music as the drummer for his band, Sobriquet.

About a year before we finished the book, the pain in my neck and brain increased markedly. Regular sleep became nearly impossible. A spinal surgeon took X-rays of my neck and diagnosed me with cervical spondylolisthesis. That's a fancy word for vertebra slippage. It causes tightness, pain, and discomfort in my neck. Unfortunately that's the same neck that my Tourette's causes me to move and shake. While surgeons can fix the problem by fusing some vertebra together, I won't be able to hold my head and neck still after the surgery. I worry that a sudden jerk could cause the fusion to break, leading to even greater problems.

It hurts. But what's new?

Many of my friends wonder if I am going to have deep brain stimulation like Jeff. Not right now. While the prospect is exciting, it's an unnecessary risk that I don't have to take. I can afford to wait until doctors refine the procedure and reduce the risks. But do I dream of the possibilities in the next ten or fifteen years? You bet I do. Even if I never have the surgery, Jeff and his amazing doctors have given me a precious gift I can never repay. He has given me a realistic belief that one day I can escape this curse and have my own Tourette's miracle. That's more than anyone else has ever given me. And for a person who often feels like he's sinking in quicksand and looking for one solid thing to hold onto, that's everything.

Since the surgery, Dr. Brian Maddux has moved his practice to Cincinnati, where he continues to treat neurological patients with the same skill and professionalism that he offered Jeff.

By far the saddest thing to happen after Jeff's surgery was the untimely death of Dr. Robert Maciunas, the architect of Jeff's miracle, on March 1, 2011. Bob Maciunas died of two aggressive and fast-moving cancers—lymphoma and renal cell carcinoma.

Maciunas's illness caused the ongoing clinical trials of DBS with Tourette's patients at University Hospitals Case Medical Center to lose steam.

The news of Maciunas's death hit everyone hard—especially Jeff. He and Debra attended the memorial service in Cleveland. There he told Maciunas's widow, Ann Failinger, how grateful he was that Maciunas had given him his life back. In turn, Failinger told Jeff how important he was to her husband, and how hard he had worked to save him. Shortly after being diagnosed with terminal cancer, Maciunas wrote this poignant good-bye to his family and friends:

> This, then, is life. I am blessed by a rich, deep, and full life; I prize being surrounded and sustained by my beloved family, my special friends, my esteemed colleagues, and my entrusted patients. I am now starting a new adventure filled both with terror and with hope. It is overwhelmingly clear how grand the provenance is that governs the web of our lives. I am sufficiently grounded to respond, " 'Tis a gift to be simple, 'tis a gift to be free," and to rejoice daily in the ennoblement of true good work, in the transcendence to be found in other people, in the meaning and the beauty of this world, and in the given mystery that is my life. I stand justified and assured of the promise of the future to come.

After Maciunas died, Jeff wrote the following, and hung it on the wall in his office under his doctor's picture.

> I am eternally grateful for every moment we spent together, and your memory will live on. Through the life you gave back to me I shall honor you, and embrace your vision, life, and passion through my actions for others, selflessness and courage. You will be missed, Dr. Maciunas. Be at peace now . . . with God at your side knowing always the difference you made in lives around the world. I will never forget you, and will always love you as you hold a very special piece of my heart. Always your pioneer, Jeff.

Acknowledgments

Jim Fussell

WHEN I WAS younger I hated it when Oscar winners thanked everyone—their wife, their parents, their dead Uncle Morty.

Then I wrote a book.

I get it now. You rarely achieve something of enduring significance by yourself. There are people who help you along the way, without whom your efforts would have been much harder, if not impossible. It's only right to acknowledge how much their assistance meant to you—no matter what anybody else thinks.

I don't have a dead Uncle Morty. But I do have a wife, so that's where I'll start.

My beautiful wife, Susan, is extraordinary by any measure. In more than thirty years of marriage she has listened to 5,479,627 things that I've read to her—or at least it seems that way. She has given me two beautiful children, rubbed my hurting neck and back more times than I can count, and always been there for me when I got stuck, didn't think I could go on, or just needed to talk. Susan, I love you and thank you for every day you've given me—and apologize for all the days I've taken from you while working on this book. I can never repay your kindness and your eternal patience—but I will try.

I also must thank my partner and my hero, Jeff Matovic. Without him there would be no miracle, and no book. Jeff is the bravest person I've ever known. Finding Jeff changed my life, gave me back the hope

251

I thought I'd lost, and inspired me to do things I had no right to be able to do. Jeff gave me a new purpose and a new belief. He has become my brother, and understands me in ways no one else can.

Of course there is one person who was not part of the story who is particularly noteworthy. This book would not have been possible without the help of a talented and special friend—my editor at the *Kansas City Star*, Sharon Hoffmann. With endless patience, a keen eye, and good cheer, she met with me week after week on her own time, giving me more than I ever expected while asking nothing in return. When I was confused about the book's structure, she gave it form and meaning. When I was in the dark, she led me to the light. She helped me when I was weak and listened to me time and again when I'm sure she had other, more important places to be. What can I say? You're amazing, Sharon, and I adore you for what you've done.

Jeff and I also are indebted to Dr. Brian Maddux for his assistance in helping us understand the complexities of deep brain stimulation surgery.

Special thank-yous also go to my amazing mother, Anita Fussell, who has helped me throughout my life more than she can ever know; to my late father, Jay Fussell, who was the finest father a son could have hoped for; to my beautiful, smart, and outstanding children, Patrick and Allison, whom I love with all my heart and would run through fire for; and to my incredible sister and brother-in-law, Nancy and John Rosenow, two of the coolest people I know. I also want to thank Dr. Maciunas's wife, Dr. Ann Failinger, whose assistance was critical in understanding her brilliant husband; and Ann Hagedorn, Rick Montgomery, Eric Adler, Matt Schofield, Laurie Mansfield, and Pam Anderson, who provided a consistent sounding board for me when I needed it most.

I also want to thank Ellen Nesselrode-Jasa of Hallmark Hall of Fame for helping me find my wonderful agent, Sharlene Martin, who tenaciously fought for this book every step of the way. Finally, a special thank-you goes to our editors and all the fine people at Chicago Review Press who believed in the worth of this project and helped make it possible.

LIKE JIM, IT drove me nuts when I watched the Oscars, Emmys, and music awards. I've not tuned in for several years because I knew I could easily get a quick rundown of the winners on the Internet or in the newspaper the next day.

I follow my partner's thought when he wrote those simple yet powerful words, "I get it now." Maybe I should have known all along that greatness achieved by others needs acknowledgment.

I've learned that with any type of accomplishment there are other people involved that had to be in the right place at the right time and the right moment to make it all come true. And now I do understand and have learned yet another valuable life lesson.

Jim and I started this project in 2004 and it has been the ride of my life in so many ways. It has allowed me to recount memories, to share a lifetime of commonalities including love, pain, anguish, humor, and tears with so many individuals who I need to thank. So, let me start.

First, my Mom, Patty, and Dad, Jim, without whom, I wouldn't be here today: there is no way to measure the amount of love, support, and dedication they have always provided. They have given endlessly to me in so many ways: physically, emotionally, spiritually, and mentally.

Never can I recall my parents putting themselves before me. Mom and Dad, for all the times you knelt by my side and prayed with me, hoping for a better tomorrow and encouraging me to be the best person I could strive to be, I can only hope to repay a fraction of what you have given me.

My childhood is filled with wonderful memories that will live on through my children all because of a woman and man who knew what they were doing was right—in love, teaching, and discipline. I grew in countless ways.

They are also very much responsible for helping me on the sleepless nights, in times of tears and triumph, sitting up all night by my hospital bed wondering what they could do to comfort me. For your greatest actions as well what some may consider small—by simply putting a cold cloth on my face or head—I cherish you both.

Your thoughts, actions, and unselfishness will always speak volumes in my mind. I will never be able to fully imagine how much you sacrificed day and night to ensure that I was safe and loved.

I will forever be indebted to your sacrifices and will try to offer you the same as our lives and relationships have only grown closer as we've moved forth. You will always be my heroes—the ones who had the healing hands, the comforting words, all the while helping me to become a better person.

Next, my brother, Steve. For watching out for my best interests when you needed to make your own strides, I am so grateful. You've helped to shape my mind and my worldly views as well as mold me into someone who understood the often underestimated value of integrity.

You provided me your shoulder more times than I can count. And on that shoulder I cried, rested, and rejoiced. Never asking for anything in return has always been a hallmark that allows me to see you as a wonderful man and father—going the extra mile to ensure stability and safety for those around you.

You've always been more than a brother. You've been my long-time mentor, teacher, healer, sounding board, and source of rational thought in times of turmoil. Your willingness to understand Tourette Syndrome allowed me to find inner strength that I didn't know I had, simply because I knew you were in my corner. You'll always have my love, admiration, respect, and never-ending thanks for all you are and continue to be.

To my wife, Debra—my rock, my lifeline, and my best friend—for your sacrifices and ability to see the inner core of me during my difficult trials and tribulations with Tourette's, I thank you. You've given me strength in times of utter despair. You rescued me from wandering into no-man's land and supported me as a man who had so much to give but without a path to follow.

You've given me beautiful children and have always made sure our family comes first. You carried my heart, soul, body, and mind through the darkness of fear and safely set me down once you knew the storm had passed and the sun was rising.

Know that you changed my life forever. I don't know how to repay you other than to let you know that I start each day with a prayer of thanks for all you've done. Each day is a new journey with you and I look forward to so many more healthy and tremendous adventures. As we watch our children grow, I ask you to stand by my side and enjoy the wonderful gifts we are so blessed to receive knowing firmly how much my heart belongs to you.

I want to send a very special thank-you to my children, Chris, Andy, Bonnie, and Mike. You're a constant reminder of the excitement and fun of being a child and keeping things simple—a lesson I believe offers parents a reminder of precious understanding and caring. You've provided me with a treasure far exceeding any price tag in the gift of being a father. Each day your smiles, successes, and joyful and playful natures bring about keen memories in which I am able treasure even more my youth and the sensations of joy they brought to my heart.

I will treasure you every day as I continue to be amazed by your strength and understanding. It's a gift I cannot describe—to watch you as you learn, change, and grow. Know always that you are my first thoughts when I awake and the ones who I say a special prayer for each night as I fall asleep. You are my life, and I couldn't be more proud of you.

Next, I thank my four grandparents and cherish the memories they gave me—all of whom I got to spend more than twenty years of my life with learning valuable lessons. Ruth and Edward Boehm and Joseph and Ann Matovic, you always provided more than I needed and were solid and grounded in your wisdom that someday I would eventually conquer my condition.

You believed in me, guided me, and instilled within me a wisdom that now I understand. Know that you are loved and missed every day as I look toward heaven and breathe the fresh air all the while knowing I will one day see you again.

To Jim Fussell, my partner, my inspiration, and my friend: the day we met was the beginning of many wonderful experiences through which we have traveled. Without you, this book was simply impossible. You've given me so much in return as we've swapped stories, learned about our "one of a kind" likenesses, and shared smiles and tears together.

Through all the calls, research, interviews, studying, late nights, planning, and laughing, I look back and see how far we've come as men and now as authors of our story—a story that started as a meeting in a hotel room and has blossomed into a brotherhood for which I am eternally grateful.

I look forward to spending the rest of our lives continuing to learn, love, and laugh together, never forgetting what it took to get us this far. The journey is just beginning. And as it has become our hallmark: Keep the Faith. You're simply amazing.

In a very special way, I thank and am forever indebted to Drs. Brian Maddux and Robert Maciunas, without whom there is no book nor my new lease of life. Your genuine care for the endurance of the human spirit lives within my heart daily. Your expertise in the field of neurology, neurosurgery, and deep brain stimulation is second to none. Thank you both for seeing the person, not the patient, as well as the courage instead of the frustration.

Next, I'd like thank University Hospitals of Cleveland (now University Hospitals Case Medical Center) for contributing its expertise to make my surgery and new life possible. In particular, I'm grateful to CEO Tom Zenty, the staff of the department of neurology, the department of neurosurgery, staff members of Tower 4 Neurological and Intensive Care Unit, and all of the nurses and staff who continue to work tirelessly to better the lives of others.

Thank you to Medtronic. Without your technology and innovative thought to care for the lives of individuals in need of electronic medical equipment, the surgery would never have taken place. Your hardware and other specific devices used in deep brain stimulation are a true measure of ingenuity and on a larger scale represent hope for people in need of these devices. Your company has provided and continues to provide hope for those in need around the globe.

Special thank-yous go to our extended families, whose insights proved most valuable to the completion of this book. Also to Dr. Ann Failinger, wife of Dr. Robert Maciunas, whose recollections and aid truly give this book meaning felt from the heart. To close friends of Jim Fussell at the *Kansas City Star* (even though we may have not have met), thank you for continuing to provide advice, counsel, and opinions to help bring this story to life.

Also thank you to Ellen Nesselrode-Jasa of Hallmark Hall of Fame for aiding us in our search for our tremendously talented agent, Sharlene Martin, who believed in our book and fought to make it the best it could possibly be.

Finally, a sincere thank-you to our editor, Jerry Pohlen, and all the dedicated people at Chicago Review Press whose belief in Jim and me and our story and passion, as well as their continued guidance made it all possible.